# HEALTHCARE CHOICES

# HEALTHCARE CHOICES

## *5 Steps to Getting the Medical Care You Want and Need*

## Archelle Georgiou, MD

ROWMAN & LITTLEFIELD
Lanham • Boulder • New York • London

Published by Rowman & Littlefield
A wholly owned subsidiary of The Rowman & Littlefield Publishing Group,
Inc.
4501 Forbes Boulevard, Suite 200, Lanham, Maryland 20706
www.rowman.com

Unit A, Whitacre Mews, 26-34 Stannary Street, London SE11 4AB

British Library Cataloguing in Publication Information Available

**Library of Congress Cataloging-in-Publication Data Available**

ISBN: 978-1-4422-6033-7 (cloth : alk. paper)
ISBN: 978-1-4422-6034-4 (electronic)

∞™ The paper used in this publication meets the minimum requirements of
American National Standard for Information Sciences Permanence of Paper
for Printed Library Materials, ANSI/NISO Z39.48-1992.

Printed in the United States of America

For my mom—my ongoing source of courage and determination

# CONTENTS

Foreword                                                              ix
    *Dan Buettner*

Acknowledgments                                                     xiii

**1** The Journey from Healthcare to Health                            1

**2** Changing Complacency to Confidence                              15

**3** The Power of Preferences over Thought Traps                     29

**4** Bring Personal Priorities to Medical Care                       51

**5** Sorting Through Alternative Care                                69

**6** Aging with Control                                             89

**7** Selecting Your Healthcare A-Team                               113

**8** Power Shopping for Health Insurance                            137

**9** Using CARES Every Day                                          159

**10** The CARES Model at a Glance                                   167

Bibliography                                                        179

Index                                                              189

About the Author                                                   193

# FOREWORD

## Dan Buettner

Not long ago, I returned from Central America with a scorching lung infection that left me listless and scared. Was it ZIKA virus, tuberculosis, or just the flu? I pondered a trip to the emergency room, but opted instead to lean on my many contacts in the healthcare industry to find a good doctor. One of the country's most famous cardiologists made a call to the Mayo Clinic to get me a lung specialist. Mayo's scheduler called me immediately, but that call just led to six more phone calls and then a dead end. Another influential friend connected me with a local specialist who, I discovered after an hour on the phone, only sees hospitalized patients. Yet another friend connected me with the University of Minnesota. They assured me that they could get me an appointment with their top pulmonologist—in three months.

Finally, after three weeks of failed attempts to get the care I needed and gasping for breath, I called Dr. Archelle Georgiou. She introduced me to CARES, the step-by-step formula she has created to help anyone evaluate their medical options and select the healthcare treatment best for them.

America's healthcare system is impossibly complex; it's based on a pay-for-services rather than a pay-for-cure model. Thousands of disconnected providers all vie for their share of the pie. Meanwhile, those of us who get sick or injured are faced with navigating a Byzantine system that often favors the bottom line over a patient's well-being. As the former CEO of one of the country's health insurance companies once told me, "We're in the business of saying no."

So our journey to getting better often begins with finding someone to say yes—and that "yes" has to come from the right provider who knows how to diagnose and treat your problem and do so effectively. A misstep along the way can result in no care, insufficient care, or, even worse, care that leaves you worse off than when you started. And stuck with a huge bill.

That's why we need this book.

Archelle's CARES model taught me how to take charge of my own healthcare. Her formula is based on five key steps: Understand Your **Condition**, Know Your **Alternatives**, **Respect** Your Preferences, **Evaluate** Your Options, and **Start** Taking Action to follow through on your healthcare decisions. Her book explained exactly how to gather accurate medical information about my lung condition and how to choose the best doctor for my care. She directed me to a number of publicly available websites to find a highly rated doctor who could treat my infection. She reminded me that you often have to advocate for the care you need. Her CARES formula ultimately put me on my path to a diagnosis and treatment by starting with a step I had completely over-looked: to call my primary care physician (who got me into a specialist the next day).

I cannot think of a more qualified healthcare expert than Archelle. During the decade that I've known her, she has served as the Chief Medical Officer of one of the nation's largest healthcare insurers. She has been an advisor to a prominent U.S. congressman, and literally millions of viewers know her in her role as the polished, uber-informed medical correspondent for KSTP-TV Eyewitness News. In 2008, Ar-chelle joined my National Geographic team to identify and explore one of the world's longest-lived areas—the so-called Blue Zone of Ikaria, Greece. There I saw her put her research, communication, and medical skills to work for a national audience. When our CNN cameraman lost his footing and plummeted from a cliff, smashing his head on the rocks below, she coolly took charge of his care. She administered first aid, oversaw his airlift to Athens, got him into the right hospital with the right surgeon, and, sixteen hours later, miraculously got him into the intensive care unit after we were told there were no available beds. Her efforts saved his life.

Not everyone is as lucky as I am—I have Archelle's number pro-grammed into my cell phone when I have a medical question. But you do have her book. Read it now and keep it on hand. I can assure you that the time will come when your health, or the health of someone you love, will take a turn for the worse. When it's your turn to find your way through the maze that is our healthcare system, Archelle's CARES formula is the guide you'll use to get to the care you need.

Dan Buettner
National Geographic Fellow and author of the *New York Times* bestsellers *The Blue Zones* and *Blue Zones Solution*

# ACKNOWLEDGMENTS

One of the most important lessons I've learned during my career is that accomplishments are never an "I" but a "we." While this book is authored under my name, there are countless family members, friends, and colleagues who inspired me, encouraged me, trusted me, and put up with me to help me get this book out of my brain and my heart and into print.

I would not have the experience to write this book had it not been for the people who believed in me early in my career. Dr. Bill McGuire, Jeannine Rivet, and Dr. Lee Newcomer understood and shared my passion for making the healthcare system easier for patients to navigate. They gave me the professional opportunity of a lifetime at United-Health Group. Thank you for having my back while we led a tumultuous sea change in the industry.

In my consulting work, I have been privileged to work with executives, innovators, clinicians, entrepreneurs, and explorers who have expanded my thinking about how to make health better and healthcare easier. I was honored to work in the Center for Health Transformation with former Speaker of the House of Representatives Newt Gingrich. Steve Bonner, former CEO of Cancer Treatment Centers of America, challenged my traditional medical mindset and introduced me to the power of evidence-based complementary and alternative medicine. Roger Holstein, former CEO of Healthgrades, ignited my deep belief that with the right tools, consumers can do the research to get to the best specialist.

Once I made a commitment to writing this book, there were very special individuals who joined the journey with me. Thank you to my agent, Helen Zimmerman, for reading my sixty-page book proposal cover to cover before our first conversation. She saw the importance of this book because she too shares a passion for improving health and healthcare. To Suzanne Staszak-Silva and Rowman & Littlefield, thank you for giving me a chance as a first-time author. Marian Deegan, my editor, brilliantly maintained my voice and intention in the writing but wasn't shy about challenging my ideas. Her quiet strength kept me accountable and confident that I'd get the manuscript done by the deadline. I absolutely could not have completed this book without her. Finally, Peter Robson gave me an open invitation to brainstorm with him. His was my right brain in this writing endeavor.

My husband, David, has been my rock for the last twenty-eight years. He's encouraged me to push myself to a level that I never dreamed was possible. My daughters—Arielle, Athena, and Zoe—gave me the confidence to write this book. They remind me, as I remind them, that there's nothing that I can't achieve.

Finally, the unsung heroes of this book are the television viewers in Minneapolis and Saint Paul who chat with me on Facebook after my news segments. Their weekly questions keep me in touch with the real challenges that real people face in our healthcare system. Only a fraction of their questions are included in these pages, but each and every one is important. They remind me that I am, first and foremost, a doctor.

# 1

# THE JOURNEY FROM HEALTHCARE TO HEALTH

If you are reading this book, you are looking for tools to make better choices for your health. You are not alone. Making healthcare decisions is hard—even for medical professionals. In an ideal world, you would sit down with the doctor best qualified to treat your condition and talk about your concerns, share information, discuss options and preferences, and agree on a treatment plan designed for you. This shared decision-making process is the goal of both consumers and healthcare professionals, but it is challenging to achieve.

The majority of people's healthcare decisions do not reflect this collaborative model, and restructuring the complexity of the healthcare system to achieve this ideal state is beyond the scope of any one person. However, each of you does have the power to participate in the decision-making process for your own health. The CARES model is a guided approach I developed to help my family and friends make medical decisions that balance the best medical treatments available with their personal priorities and preferences. This book allows me to share the model and the tools with you so that you too can get the healthcare you want, need, and deserve.

## LESSONS FROM IKARIA

In 2009, my career reflected a breadth of medical, insurance, and media experience as a healthcare advocate. I'd been a practicing physician,
the chief medical officer for the country's largest health insurer, a con-
sultant to healthcare businesses, a member of the media reporting on
health issues, and, last (but certainly not least), the mother of three
young women and the wife of an actively practicing gastroenterologist.

However, the passion and defining experiences captured in this
book unfolded on the tiny island of Ikaria. On this windswept, ninety-
eight-square-mile Greek refuge in the northern Aegean Sea, a population of about 8,500 inhabitants live in homes camouflaged to protect
them from the pirates of days gone by. Over the centuries, Ikarians had
mysteriously developed a lifestyle that protected them from the ravages
of old age as well as rapacious raids by buccaneers. In April 2009,
explorer and bestselling author Dan Buettner, with funding from the
National Geographic Expeditions Council and the National Institute on
Aging, asked me to join him on an international research trip to identify
"Blue Zones," small pockets of communities populated with an excep-
tionally high percentage of people living to one hundred years of age or
more. Dan had already explored four other Blue Zones; Ikaria was the
final stop. I was intrigued. My Greek heritage and my passion for improving healthcare could not resist an opportunity to explore clues to
longevity in a country that I considered a second home.

In Ikaria, we joked that "people forget to die." The islanders live into
their nineties at several times the rate of Americans. Ikarians had significantly lower instances of cancer, cardiovascular disease, and diabetes—
during our trip, we met only one individual with even a hint of dementia.[1] The lifestyle findings we identified in Ikaria were fascinating, and
consistent with Dan's observations in Okinawa, Japan; Sardinia, Italy;
Nicoya, Costa Rica; and Loma Linda, California. Ikarians eat a plant-
based diet, and virtually everything served at their tables comes from
their own garden because importing food to this outlying island is expensive and unpredictable. They also "move naturally," as Dan says.
Ikarians don't go to the gym; they get a good workout simply by walking
the rugged terrain during their daily activities. However, their longevity
secret goes beyond diet and exercise. Ikarians maintain a sense of purpose. They don't retire—they rewire and maintain responsibilities on

their family farms well into old age. Finally, these generous hospitable islanders remain actively connected to friends and family.

For a Johns Hopkins–trained physician, these observations alone would have been enough to open my eyes to a broader definition of what it means to be healthy. But a specific and dramatic event brought my Ikarian experience into focus and shaped my current view about the difference between health and healthcare. During our two-week stay, our activities were being filmed for a series of live satellite interviews with CNN's Anderson Cooper. Our Greek videographer, Emmanuel Tambakakis, was superb, and had earned an international reputation for doing whatever it took to get the perfect shot. One of our last shoots took place in thermal waters at the base of a steep rocky cliff. Emmanuel found his perfect shot looking down from the edge of the cliff. While setting up the camera and satellite cables, the ground beneath his feet crumbled. He lost his balance and fell, smashing against boulders and tumbling fifty feet to the middle of the cliff face. From the beach, I heard screams for help from Dan and our satellite technician and sprinted up the precipice to reach Emmanuel. He was unconscious when I reached him. His face was smeared with blood and rocks; his eyelids were blue and swollen. As I carefully checked to see whether he had a pulse and was breathing, I noticed a trickle of clear fluid from his left ear. This was a telltale sign of an epidural hematoma—an accumulation of blood between the brain and the skull caused by a ruptured artery. To survive, Emmanuel needed emergency treatment within hours.

Ikaria had no hospital or emergency room. The most advanced technology on the island was an x-ray machine. For emergencies like this, people are transported via helicopter to Samos, the neighboring island, and then flown to Athens for hospital care. It was dusk, and too dark to safely make the thirty-minute jump to Samos. The Greek medical evacuation system was paralyzed by its own bureaucracy, and there were no commercial flights to Athens until morning. Emmanuel was dying.

Fortunately for Emmanuel, he had a resource that Ikarians do not: the power and international influence of CNN. Our contacts at the network's Atlanta-based office responded to our call, communicating and coordinating Emmanuel's care nonstop for thirty-six hours. As I sat on the hillside beside my unconscious friend, our producer handed me the phone and I found myself talking to one of the top neurosurgeons in the United States who coached me through the steps I needed to take to stabilize Emmanuel. CNN convinced the Greek government to send a jet to Ikaria and a C-27J Spartan military plane arrived two hours later. Emmanuel underwent life-saving emergency neurosurgery in Athens that night. Thanks to the heroic efforts and persuasive global connections of our CNN team, Emmanuel made a full recovery.

In the weeks and months following, I found myself replaying the accident and my own emotional reactions to it. I was frightened—and confused. What would happen if an Ikarian fell from that cliff, without access to CNN resources? Death was almost a foregone conclusion. How did the Ikarians have such extraordinary health, as evidenced by their longevity, in the *absence* of a sophisticated healthcare system? The island had probably lost a good number of people to traumatic injuries, yet the island's overall health statistics far exceeded those of Americans with access to the most advanced medical resources. For the first time in my career, I realized that *health* and *healthcare* are not synonymous.

This insight took me beyond Dan's published findings that diet, exercise, purpose, and family/social connections can stretch one's years. As a physician steeped in my Greek heritage, I came to my own hypothesis about Ikarian longevity: Ikarians have health without advanced healthcare because they have been forced to be self-reliant and look first to themselves—not a doctor—for care. When they have a twinge of pain or a bothersome symptom, Ikarians' first instinct is to patiently trust their body's self-healing ability. A common expression on the island is "tha perasi" or "it will pass." When ailments persist, they try "indigenous" home remedies. Skin rash? Take a dip in the sea. Stomachache? Drink an herbal tea. Knee pain? Apply warm towels and avoid walking uphill.

Worrisome or persistent symptoms typically prompt Ikarians to pop in and visit the local pharmacist for advice before they consult a doctor—a clinic visit with the area's sole primary care doctor can be a daylong ordeal.[2] Ikarians' self-reliance continues even while they are under the doctor's care. The primary care physician currently assigned to western Ikaria told me that Ikarians adhere to their treatment plan and are 90 to 100 percent compliant with their prescription medications. Their motivation? Avoiding a trip to Athens for more advanced care. When Ikarians face a decision about treatment for a serious illness, they discuss and weigh all their options—they know that surgery or other advanced care will require significant time, cost, and complex logistics. Geographic isolation has forced Ikarians to actively participate in decisions regarding their health.

I am struck by the contrast between the Ikarian approach to healthcare and the culture of care in the United States. Americans, in general, are far from self-reliant when it comes to their health. I will boldly go further and describe our nation's approach to care as passively dependent. When Americans experience something that just "doesn't feel right," the reflex behavior is to see a doctor who can "find it and fix it." According to a 2012 survey by the Centers for Disease Control, there were almost one billon physician office visits in the United States in a single year.[3] The most common reason for an office visit? Cough. When I've asked people why they sought medical advice for common cold symptoms, the usual response is, "I just wanted to make sure that I wasn't missing anything since I'm not a doctor." Ikarians do not presume to have the knowledge of a physician, but they do have the self-confidence to make choices about when to get care, where to get care, and what care they prefer. Americans, on the other hand, tend to lack this self-confidence. They depend on medical professionals, passively ceding control of their healthcare decisions to doctors, insurers, hospitals, and other authorities within the system.

My observations in Ikaria brought me to the belief that there is a better way to achieve health in America—without moving to a remote island, living a rustic lifestyle, and growing your own food. You can achieve better health by replacing passive "fix me" behaviors with self-reliant ones—new habits that keep you actively involved in your own care. New habits require new tools.

I am encouraging you to make a significant change in the way you approach your own health and healthcare. I realize that cultivating new habits is no easy task, and committing to change is not easy. This is why I would like to share with you my own journey through change that starts with the stories of my immigrant family's determination to make a better life. Their courage inspired me, as I hope it will inspire you.

November 8 has always been a special day. It was my father's nameday, and in Greek families, namedays are more important than birthdays. In our very traditional home, this meant an annual open house for my dad, complete with mountains of stuffed grape leaves, platters of triangle-shaped cheese pies, and trays of honey-drenched baklava. The party was also an opportunity for my dad, a master tailor, to take a short break from his seventy-hour work week. He owned a dry cleaners in downtown Baltimore, and for the forty-plus years that he was in business, his primary goal was earning enough to pay for our college educations—in cash.

November 8 was also the day my mother arrived in the Port of New York in 1951. She left Greece as a young woman of nineteen, wearing white ankle socks and a dress sewn from a potato sack. Seven years of hardship and hunger—four years during World War II and three more years during the Greek Civil War—gave my mother the courage to leave her parents and six siblings to build a new life in the United States under the auspices of President Truman's Displaced Persons Act of 1948. Each year, on the anniversary of her arrival, my mom retells the story of her journey. Determined to find the U.S. sponsor she needed to sign her visa application, she found her way to Athens. A hotel lobby was her home for two nights until she secured a sponsor and her visa. She negotiated a loan for the eight hundred dollars she needed to pay for her boat ticket, proudly reminding us that she paid back every penny, just as she promised she would.

Each year, my parents' stories rekindle my admiration for their conviction that they could and would find a new and better way to live their lives. As my family gathered to celebrate my graduation from The John Hopkins University School of Medicine in 1986, my medical degree opened the door to my new life as a physician. In ways I didn't realize at the time, their vision of a brighter future would continue to inspire my professional journey.

For five years, I practiced internal medicine in San Ramon, a suburb in the San Francisco Bay Area. This affluent community was home to the corporate headquarters of Chevron, 24-Hour Fitness, General Electric's global software center, and the West Coast office of AT&T. With a median family income of about $100,000, my patients were primarily middle-aged, well-educated women with the intention and the resources to take care of their health.

My practice grew and flourished. I shared idyllic office space with my husband's gastroenterology practice. Our daughters visited often, watching Looney Tunes videos on the procedure room monitors when David wasn't doing a sigmoidoscopy. I was elected chairman of the

Department of Internal Medicine. On the surface, my career seemed perfect. Nevertheless, over time, a math equation had taken shape in my mind. If I followed the traditional path, seeing fifteen patients each day, every day, for the next thirty years, I'd have a medical impact on about 100,000 people over the course of my career. Would that be enough? Would I be making enough of a difference in healthcare? Should I take steps to change the numbers in the equation—to make more of a difference? Unlike my parents, there was no hardship to force my hand. I had an engraved nameplate on my office door, a beautiful medical office, a happy, fulfilling life, and no compelling incentive to change.

Then, in one day, with one patient and one test result, all that changed.

As my husband and I practiced medicine in 1993, the healthcare industry was experiencing the dawn of a managed care revolution. Access to healthcare was in the midst of "a rapid shift from traditional indemnity plans to health maintenance organizations (HMOs) and other network plans, for large and small businesses alike," reported Susan Marquis and Stephen Long, senior economists at the RAND Corporation, a nonprofit institution that helps improve policy and decision-making through research and analysis.[4] This was a period when managed care companies had none of the checks and balances now in place—and we were practicing in California, a state infamous for its stringent controls in this arena.

My colleagues and I struggled with the bureaucratic hassles of managed care and speculated about how these relatively new types of insurance plans—with their myriad rules and restrictions—had unsettling potential to interfere with our ability to deliver high quality care to patients.

Worrisome potential turned into grave reality when a patient named Cindy visited my office for a routine Pap smear. This test detects cervical cancer as well as changes in cervical cells that suggest the development of cancer in the future. Women who've had a Pap smear know that it is a painless procedure that takes less than a minute. I used a tiny plastic spatula and small brush, gently swiping the surface and opening of the cervix to collect cells for analysis by a pathology lab.

I'd performed this procedure hundreds of times in my practice. Pap smears had identified cancer in a few patients. Many more patients had "atypical cells" requiring a follow-up procedure, a colposcopy, to look for microscopic changes in the cervical tissue. But *none* of these women bled during the Pap smear test itself.

Cindy bled profusely. This suggested only a few possibilities. One was that I had used too much force and traumatized her cervix. Possible, but unlikely. I was experienced and she reported no pain. The other possibility raised an alarm in my head: "Okay, Cindy's tissue is so fragile and raw that a light scraping causes bleeding. Something is wrong."

I fully expected the Pap smear result to be abnormal. During her visit, I forewarned Cindy that I was concerned and that I'd be referring her to a gynecologist as soon as the pathology report was available. Three days later, Cindy's Pap smear results came back normal. I was perplexed. My first reaction was that there'd been a mistake; maybe the blood obscured the sample and made it difficult for the pathologist to detect the abnormal cervical cells that I was certain were present. Or maybe Cindy's Pap smear sample was mislabeled and the "normal" cells were from another patient. I thought back to the bleeding during the procedure, relied on my clinical judgment, and referred Cindy to a gynecologist—after dutifully completing the HMO referral form. In my referral, I described the bleeding that occurred during her exam and wrote: "Suspect abnormal tissue. Needs colposcopy." I attached the pathology report and assumed my rationale would be sufficient for the HMO to approve the procedure.

Several days later the gynecologist (who was also a friend) called and said, "Archelle, I can't do a colposcopy on your patient. With a normal Pap smear, the insurance company won't consider it medically necessary and won't pay for the procedure."

Medical necessity guidelines are insurance company rules that require treating physicians to justify the clinical rationale for performing any procedure. If a doctor's rationale does not meet the healthplan's guidelines, the HMO or managed care medical director can deny coverage for the service.

"The Pap smear may be normal, but the patient's cervix isn't normal," I replied. "I've never had a patient bleed profusely during a routine gyn exam. We need to treat the patient, not the test result." I couldn't let laboratory evidence trump clinical evidence: in this case, friable, bleeding tissue. "Please. Just do it," I said. "If you don't get reimbursement for it by the HMO, I'll personally pay you for the procedure."

He did the colposcopy and the results confirmed my concerns: Cindy had invasive uterine cancer. One week later she had a radical hysterectomy. Fortunately, Cindy did well. For me, the event fundamentally changed the course of my career. I saw with my own eyes how an HMO's decision could cause delays in care, inadequate care, or even death.

Cindy's medical situation inspired me to start my own journey to change the system and to act on that math equation in my mind. I had protected Cindy, but I wanted to protect the millions of others whose care was being unnecessarily denied. I made it my mission to try to unravel the harmful rules that managed care imposes on doctors, patients, and hospitals and craft a more collaborative way for doctors and insurance companies to work together. To my colleagues, my vision for eliminating the frustrating bureaucracy that held us back from practicing good medicine was a pipe dream. But with my parents' determination fueling me, I was convinced that there was a better model.

Within a year of Cindy's diagnosis, my own "visa" to begin the journey to a better healthcare system materialized. I was invited to attend a series of meetings at Cigna Healthcare of California. Eventually, I was offered a part-time position as an associate medical director. It felt like a small door had opened. I was in the right place to be to achieve my hope for change—inside a health insurance company.

My primary responsibility as an associate medical director was to review doctors' requests for expensive tests and procedures and to either approve or deny them based on the company's "evidence-based" guidelines. More than once I found myself on the phone with a doctor whose rationale for a surgery, submitted on a form, didn't meet the company's definition of "medically necessary." I was performing the very same review that made me indignant when I was practicing, but I approached it differently. In my role, I had the authority to deny the request, but I also had the authority to override the company's guidelines. My approach was to give the physician an opportunity to explain his or her clinical reasoning so that I could stamp "APPROVE." I approved the vast majority of these requests, but I was one medical director in one insurance company; the rest of the industry was continuing to deny care and the cynicism and frustration of physicians dealing with managed care continued.

My former colleagues in San Ramon asked how I was enjoying the "dark side" of medicine. I loved it. Despite the challenges, my new position provided me with an opportunity to see healthcare through unique lenses. As an insurance insider, I had data on the healthcare costs for an entire population broken down by detailed service categories—inpatient, outpatient, physician, pharmacy, and mental health. I had charts and graphs on hospital admission patterns. And I had access to approval and denial data—not anecdotes—as well as customer satisfaction (often dissatisfaction) results.

The data I saw proved that managed care's approval and denial "Mother may I" process wasn't effective. It was not controlling costs, was expensive to administer, made doctors angry, and put patients at risk. Over time, research supported my point of view. In 1998, Dr. Robert Blendon, professor of health policy and political analysis at Harvard University, published the results of a survey in *Health Affairs*. His findings came as no surprise to me: 59 percent of Americans said that managed care plans made it harder for sick people to see medical specialists, half (51 percent) said that managed care had decreased the quality of care for people who are sick, and the majority (55 percent) said that they were at least "somewhat worried" that if they were sick, their healthplan would be more concerned about saving money than about providing them with the best medical treatment.[5]

With the support of senior medical directors around the country, I started constructing a process to bypass the "Mother may I" model. The timing wasn't right for Cigna to adopt such progressive thinking. Implementation stalled.

During my eighteen months with Cigna, my work caught the eye of a competitor, UnitedHealthcare of California. In 1995, I went to work for them.[6] Two years later, our family moved to Minneapolis, the home of UnitedHealthcare's corporate office, so that I could take on a broader role as a National Medical Director.

UnitedHealthcare's CEO, Dr. William McGuire, was a physician himself. He supported a more physician-friendly, patient-centric company culture. In 1994, the company boldy discontinued the "gatekeeper model" so that members could see a specialist without a referral. However, medical necessity requirements were still being imposed—the same rules that could have led to Cindy's demise. Dr. McGuire frequently questioned the clinical and business value of the approval and denial process—but his team hadn't developed an alternative.

I saw a window of opportunity to pilot test the concepts I had developed at Cigna in March 1999. Within three months, the results of the pilot were breathtaking. Patient readmissions dropped. Physicians were astounded and delighted by our collaborative approach to their care requests. Our own internal healthplan nurses and physicians welcomed their redefined mission to manage care—instead of denying it. Though it was still too early to fully calculate the financial results, it was clear that our pilot's revolutionary coordinated care approach was the right thing to do.

Later that year, I was promoted to Chief Medical Officer (CMO) and took on the clinical oversight for twenty-six healthplan medical management units providing care for seventeen million Americans. As the CMO, I was no longer responsible for *administering* the company's policies. My new position provided me with the influence to *change* the company's policies, and in October 1999, UnitedHealthcare eliminated the "Mother may I" process. In its place, we reorganized our company's 1,500-plus nurses and medical directors under a new "Care Coordination" model that worked *with* doctors and hospitals, not against them, to get patients the care they needed.

November 8, that charmed date in my family's history, was poised to deliver another momentous event to add to our family's chronicles. On November 8, 1999, a front-page story by Charles Ornstein of the *Dallas Morning News* brought national attention to the success of our Care Coordination model.[7] Within hours, United's elimination of medical necessity review was the lead story on every major newscast; by the next morning it was the front-page story in newspapers across the country. Our story generated some 263 *million* media impressions. The American Medical Association, consumer advocacy groups, and even President Bill Clinton applauded us for our policy change. The media attention mirrored the groundbreaking nature of our move. It was a wake-up call to other insurers that they too should loosen their policies. UnitedHealthcare was at the forefront of a historic, dramatic sea change in managed care.

When Cindy's plight prompted me to actively take up the challenge of "medical necessity" guidelines, I never imagined that my work would drive a national change in healthcare. As the architect of a revolution in the healthcare industry in 1999, I was immensely proud and thought my work was done. It wasn't until I traveled to Ikaria that I realized it wasn't enough to change the way insurance managed medical care. I wanted to revolutionize our nation's culture of care—the personal approach to managing our own health and healthcare.

You may find it daunting to contemplate taking active responsibility for the management of your care, but my experience on Ikaria has convinced me that this is not merely possible—it is your right and responsibility as a healthcare consumer. I want to use my knowledge to provide you with the tools you need to make choices that protect your health and help you access the best resources our healthcare system has to offer. You can take the first step by learning how to make informed healthcare choices.

Throughout my career, and especially during my last nine years as a health expert on KSTP-TV, I've helped thousands of friends and television viewers struggling with health-related issues. "Do I need to go to the doctor?" "Should I agree to another round of chemotherapy?" "What's the best insurance to buy?" The questions span a vast range from simple to complex and from clinical to administrative. What they seem to have in common is confusion about *how* to make a healthcare decision. When I reply, I don't diagnose, prescribe, or treat. I educate people about the facts and issues they need to consider in order to make the right choice—for them.

Answering viewers' questions is a highlight of my week and helps me stay connected to the community. But the math equation that haunted me as a physician is still in my mind. How many individual questions can I answer over the remainder of my career? How many would be enough for me to be making the most valuable difference in healthcare? There are so many people desperate to have someone guide them through our dizzyingly complex healthcare system. It is my hope that this book can help them—and you—find the direction needed.

I wrote this book to lay out a simple, structured approach to making healthcare decisions. The CARES model I describe is the process I rely on when I answer viewers' questions or have a friend say, "Can I ask you to put your doctor hat on?" In some situations, the clinical issues are important. I draw on my medical knowledge to answer those questions. More frequently, however, my advice doesn't require a medical degree. The clinical information is straightforward, and other dimensions, like values, preferences, convenience, and cost, are the issues I help people sort through.

My CARES approach to healthcare is very different from the approach most Americans take when making healthcare decisions. Using these tools is not as easy as "find it and fix it." But learning to use my CARES approach in your own decision making will give you healthcare independence. Using CARES doesn't mean being your own doctor or rejecting the advice of clinical professionals. It does mean having the self-confidence to identify and evaluate all your options so that you can be an active partner in your own health, advocate for yourself, and ultimately make the right healthcare decisions *for you*.

My dad sat at a sewing machine for seventy hours a week. My mother slept in a hotel lobby for two nights to get the visa she needed to realize her dream of a new life in the United States. Their courage inspired me to do what it takes for the chance to live a better life. Their determination was the fuel for my journey through healthcare—from Johns Hopkins to UnitedHealthcare to Ikaria to these pages where I have compiled tools for you to use to take charge of your health.

I hope my story will inspire you to reconnect with the values that shaped your family's American dream. You too have a family history that is rooted in optimism and determination. It is my hope that CARES will help you claim responsibility for your health so that you can thrive in pursuit of your personal dreams for a better life.

Tap your legacy as I did, and harness it to begin the journey to better health and the excellent healthcare you and your family deserve.

## NOTES

1. Dan Buettner's work was published in the bestselling *Blue Zones: Lessons for Living Longer From the People Who've Lived the Longest* (Washington, DC: National Geographic Society, 2008).

2. In 2009, there were two primary care physicians assigned to the western side of Ikaria. In July 2015, there was one. The number of physicians fluctuates with the economy and the number of physicians willing to move to the island.

3. "National Center for Health Statistics," Centers for Disease Control and Prevention, http://www.cdc.gov/nchs/fastats/physician-visits.htm.

4. M. S. Marquis and S. H. Long, "Trends in Manager Care and Competition, 1993–1997," *Health Affairs* 18, no. 6 (1999): 75–88, doi:10.1377/hlthaff.18.6.75. http://content.healthaffairs.org/content/18/6/75.full.pdf?origin=publication_detail.

5. R. J. Blendon, "Understanding the Managed Care Backlash," *Health Affairs*, no. 4 (1998): 80–94.

6. I was hired by MetraHealth in March 1995. MetraHealth was acquired by UnitedHealthcare in October 1995.

7. Charles Ornstein, "UnitedHealth to Let Doctors Set Treatments," *Dallas Morning News*, November 8, 1999.

# 2

# CHANGING COMPLACENCY TO CONFIDENCE

**F**acebook Questions

*Andrea: My daughter woke up with a high temp this morning, bad cough (flu-like symptoms). What can doctors do if you go see them with flu-like symptoms? Or can I do the same stuff at home?*

*Dr. Georgiou: Most kids will do fine at home. Treat the symptoms just like you would for any other cold or flu. Reasons to get medical care are if your child has shortness of breath, looks dehydrated, has persistent vomiting, or a fever that is increasing over the next few days rather than decreasing.*

*Marsha: I think my immune system needs a boost. Every time some-one sick is around me, I get sick. What can I do to help with low immunity?*

*Dr. Georgiou: Your "symptoms" don't necessarily mean you have low immunity. But there are lifestyle behaviors that can decrease the risk of getting sick from what are likely to be viral infections. These are pretty basic but important because they work: good hand hy-giene, especially if you are around someone who is sick; getting enough sleep (FYI, sleep deprivation alters the immune system) and regular exercise. Also, while there's not a lot of data to support it, many doctors recommend a multivitamin.*

*Marsha: Yeah, I really don't get enough sleep. Well, that helped.*

These are two questions I received following my weekly TV segment "Inside Your Health" as medical expert for KSTP-TV in Minneapolis. I get dozens of questions like these through the station's Facebook page[1] as well as on my fan page, Archelle MD,[2] each time I appear on the evening news. I cite these in particular not because their medical problems were so confounding; in fact, 10 percent of the inquiries I get are related to confusion about whether symptoms are "just a cold" versus the flu. Nor do I begin this book with these questions because my responses broke new medical ground. My answers probably offer the same information an intern right out of medical school would be able to share.

I share these questions because I think they are good examples of the problems embedded in the fabric of the American cultural belief system. Namely:

- Too many people have a basic lack of information about how to truly "take care" of themselves, despite having so many resources at their fingertips to educate themselves.
- People have significant insecurities about managing their symptoms, let alone initiating preventive measures.
- Because of the previous two factors, people reflexively turn to doctors for answers that they could find themselves.
- Finally, in the great fast food, One Minute Manager, instant enlightenment tradition Americans are so enamored with, they simply (simply?) want a quick diagnosis and a quicker fix.

Do these advertising tag lines for cold meds ring a bell?

"Fast-acting Advil."
"Anacin, fast pain relief."
"Sucrets . . . for fast sore throat and cough relief."
"Alka Seltzer. . . . Fast relief from your worst cold and flu symptoms."

Perhaps you will recognize some of these phrases from America's $60.5 billion weight loss market,[3] which is fueled by the insatiable desire for a silver bullet to get thin . . . fast:

"Alli: . . . results in the first two weeks."

"Garcinia Cambogia: . . . Burn fat faster. All with just two capsules a day."

ATX-101: "New Magic Injection to Get Rid of Your Double Chin."[4]

Pharmaceutical manufacturers are more than happy to feed the demand of those who want "fast relief." In fact, when some companies develop a product that does not seem to treat a known symptom, they will "manufacture" a treatable condition. Such was the famous case with sildenafil, synthesized by British chemists at Pfizer, hoping it would treat hypertension and angina. Clinical trials suggested the drug had little effect on angina, but it could induce penile erections. Thus Viagra was born and approved by the FDA in 1998. It was the first oral treatment for what is commonly known as impotence, but Pfizer created a new medical diagnosis: erectile dysfunction. Viagra's blockbuster sales spawned the development of similar medications, and annual U.S. sales of Viagra, Cialis, and Levitra now average about two billion dollars.[5]

Drug manufacturers also capitalize on complications of medications that are overprescribed. In 2014, almost two million Americans abused or were dependent on prescription opioids, and more than fourteen thousand people died from overdoses.[6] As Congress declares opioid addiction a national epidemic, pharmaceutical companies see it as a profit-making opportunity. Drugs designed to combat the "opioid-induced constipation" caused by narcotic painkillers are projected to generate $561 billion in sales by 2019.[7] The "find it and fix it" mentality pervades the marketplace, and the high-speed ability of technology serves to further fuel Americans' thirst for immediacy. That, in turn, increases the expectation of a cure, or at least answers to questions about what's going wrong within their bodies—now!

This is America's culture of care, but it's not working to our advantage. The consequence of the demand for fast answers to complicated health matters is the endless demand for tests, diagnostics, and pharmaceuticals. U.S. patients receive ninety-one MRI exams per 100,000 people, compared to fewer than fifty exams per 100,000 in five other reporting countries.[8] Despite all this healthcare, costing the nation $3.3 trillion each year, Americans don't experience better health.[9] On nearly all indicators of mortality, survival, and life expectancy, the United States consistently ranks at or near the bottom among high-income countries.

How did we get here?

It's easy to point fingers and simply assume that patients don't want to take personal responsibility for their care. I remember being in clinical practice and getting quietly frustrated when patients swung by the emergency room on their way home from work because they were worried they might be coming down with a cold. Didn't they know to drink fluids, use over-the-counter cold remedies, and wash their hands? It's also easy to point fingers at doctors and assume that we are prescription writers and procedure orderers who don't take the time to communicate with patients about all their treatment options. And it's convenient to vilify health insurance companies by suggesting that they put profit in front of patients.

How we got here—how we developed our attitude toward health and healthcare—is not anyone's fault. It's everyone's. America's culture of health evolved over the last 240 years and is woven into the nation's fabric. I see eight critical threads in that fabric.

1. Core values.

Generally and even historically speaking, Americans are very good at following rules. They stay within the lines on highways, they fill out tax forms by April 15, they "honor their fathers and mothers." Indeed, the religious beliefs and convictions of the Founding Fathers—a group of men who represented by and large the Christian faiths that some now call Fundamentalist—formed the foundations of the American value system. Those values have transcended the walls of their originating religious institutions and have created the framework of a society that continues to reinforce the need, actually the obligation, to ask for permission—permission from parents, teachers, political leadership, pastors, and professional superiors, including physicians. Results from the World Values Survey support these statements. They show that the United States is one of the highest-scoring countries on the Traditional Values dimension, which emphasizes religiosity, national pride, respect for authority, and obedience.[10]

There is, of course, a great irony in all this. Americans—from the land of the free and the home of the brave, a democratic society of free speech and independent-minded men and women encompassing the early Pilgrims, the frontiersmen, the innovators and explorers, and the entrepreneurs and creative forces of today—are not followers at all. Yet when it comes to our most precious commodity, our own health, many of us are like sheep following whatever our doctors and insurance companies and other medical care providers tell us to do and not to do about our health.

## Facebook Question

*Vanessa: Does a doctor ever have the right to yell at a patient?*

*Dr. Georgiou: Absolutely not. Never. If your doctor is yelling at you, fire him/her and find a new doctor who you can have a mutually respectful relationship with.*

2. Language.

The language you use to identify yourself and define your relationships influences how you interact, how you behave, and what you expect of each other. When you refer to yourself as a "patient," you assume that role, a role with implications you may not realize. A paper published in the *British Medical Journal* explains that "the word 'patient' conjures up a vision of quiet suffering, of someone lying in a bed waiting for the doctor to come by and give of his or her skill, and of an unequal relationship between the user of healthcare services and the provider."[11] Patients address their physicians as "Doctor," while the physician usually calls patients by their first name. And the term "doctor/patient relationship" is much more common than "patient/doctor relationship." These communication norms hardly encourage a partnership, but rather reinforce a hierarchical relationship between those who provide care and those who receive it.

## Archelle's Insider Tip

*Small, nuanced changes in the wording you use during interactions with doctors can make a big difference in how you view your role. So . . .*

- *When you call to make an appointment, don't say, "I am Dr. Jones' patient and would like to make an appointment." This phrasing suggests that Dr. Jones has all the power. Instead say, "I see Dr. Jones and would like to make an appointment."*
- *Upon meeting new doctors, if they enter the room and introduce themselves as "Dr. Jones," respond with: "Brad Jones? Nice to*

*meet you. I am Archelle Georgiou." Acknowledging their first name reminds you and him that you are both human.*

- *In a follow-up visit, continue to use first names. Trust me, it's not disrespectful. In fact, they are unlikely to notice because it is their name. Infusing informality into the relationship can naturally foster more informal and open communication.*
- *They will inevitably ask, "How are you?" and expect you to launch into a diatribe about the medical reason for the visit. Instead, first share something positive about your day, your family, an upcoming vacation. Then ask the doctor, "How are you doing?" Connecting on a social level reminds both of you that you have lives and interests outside of this clinical interaction.*

3. Regulatory definition of "care."

State licensing requirements for health providers—physicians, nurses, pharmacists, mental health practitioners, etc.—and facilities help assure that patients are treated by qualified and competent professionals in safe environments. However, these regulatory standards have inadvertently hijacked the definition of "care." How? By limiting the responsibility and reimbursement for care only to licensed clinicians who perform services and procedures worthy of reimbursement by insurance companies. The consequence? A healthcare system and a culture that doesn't place value on self-care or the care/support for health and wellness provided by family, friends, and community.

4. Employee benefits.

Receiving employment-based health insurance benefits is a phenomenon that evolved when legislation passed in 1939 excluded health insurance benefits as taxable [12] income. In 1954, tax laws changed again to allow employers to deduct health insurance benefits as a business expense. [13]

Currently, about 60 percent of Americans with health insurance receive these benefits through an employer's group plan. Employees view health insurance benefits as an important component of their compensation because employers typically pay for a majority of the premium. While nice for the paycheck, this perk comes at a price. Employees are shielded from being healthcare consumers because they rely on their employers' priorities and judgment instead of their own to select insurance carriers, deductible and premium amounts, and medical benefits that are covered. The unintended consequence? Employees' dependence on employers for access to healthcare fuels complacency regarding the cost of insurance and snowballs into helplessness toward identifying and advocating for the best and highest quality of care. How complacent? Despite the availability of free online data, studies show that people spend more time researching their next refrigerator purchase than they do researching their doctor or hospital.[14] I'm going to show you how to do this research in chapter 7.

Archelle's Insider Tip

*Your insurance coverage is a contract between you and the insurer. You are responsible for knowing the rules, what's covered, and, most importantly, what's not covered. Before enrolling in any health insurance plan—whether it's through your employer, a health insurance exchange, or through an insurance broker—make sure to:*

- *Ask for the Evidence of Coverage for your plan. It may also be called a "Summary Plan Description." It outlines what you can expect from the insurance company and what they expect of you.*
- *Read the section titled "Coverage Limits and Exclusions." This is the most critical section to read because it lists healthcare services that are not covered—that is, will not be paid by the insurer, even if you are terminally ill.*
- *Remember: you have a choice. If you feel one particular plan is too limited for your health needs, the Affordable Care Act, through the Health Insurance Exchanges, gives you the option of exploring other healthplan coverage.*

5. "Managed" care.

The growth of HMOs and managed care in the United States was spurred by the Health Maintenance Organization Act of 1973. The goal was to ensure that healthcare coverage included more comprehensive benefits at a more affordable cost than traditional insurance. Indeed, the attractiveness of managed care plans for consumers and employers has resulted in 44 percent of Americans receiving their healthcare through HMOs and other types of managed care organizations. But here's the catch: insurance companies keep premiums affordable by imposing various controls that literally "manage care." These controls force patients and their doctors to first contact the managed care company for approval to receive care, whether it's to see a specialist, get physical therapy, or have surgery. So insurance company–salaried doctors and nurses determine the "medical necessity" of treatments—without ever seeing patients themselves. If they decide a doctor's services are not medically necessary, insurance doesn't pay.

In a culture that already bows down to the authority of physicians, these permission-seeking rules require obedience with an even higher authority, namely the insurance company controlling the purse strings. Sadly, it's not just consumers who passively accept what the HMO tells them they need. The maddening time drain of insurance bureaucracy involved in appealing a managed care denial has discouraged physicians from advocating on behalf of their patients. Except in the most egregious situations, clinicians tend to acquiese and accommodate insurers' decisions.

## Facebook Question

*Anonymous: My brother was seriously injured in an accident, severing his spinal cord, about 4 1/2 weeks ago. He is now paralyzed from his waist down. He spent seventeen days in ICU and has been in rehab at HealthSouth and making great progress. His insurance, United Health Care, informed him they would not cover any additional days since he is only receiving "custodial" care. I am more than frustrated because his incredible progress and positive outlook is now deteriorating. What can I do? I am very unfamiliar with resources in this area.*

*Dr. Georgiou: Managed care companies have to comply with strict regulations. Your first step should be to get a physical or electronic copy of the insurance company's denial letter for continued rehabilitation. The insurer can't simply deny ongoing care by verbal communication. They have to issue a letter, explain their rationale, and cite the section in the Evidence of Coverage that defines the benefit limits for Inpatient Rehabilitative Care that supports their decision.*

6. Healthcare reimbursement.

Another control instituted by managed care companies is their method for paying doctors. To be contracted as an "in network" provider, doctors agree to accept a discount on their rates. How much of a discount? On average, managed care organizations reimburse doctors 50 to 60 percent of their fees. Due to the discounts they agree to, doctors compress the time with each patient in order to fit more visits and procedures into their day to compensate for the lost income per patient. Based on data from the most recent National Ambulatory Medical Care Survey, the average amount of time a patient spends with a physician during an office visit is 20.8 minutes.[15] While this is an improvement from the seventeen-minute visit average in the 1990s, this relatively brief interaction is not conducive to a relationship that allows people to be actively engaged partners in their care. Surveys show that people rate the relationship with a physician only second in importance to the relationship with their spouse. However, imagine only having one or two 20.8-minute encounters with a spouse or life partner twice a year. What kind of relationship would that be?

### Archelle's Insider Tip

*Does this sound familiar? You call to schedule a "follow-up appointment" with your doctor to get her opinion on several symptoms continuing to bother you. Well organized, you make a list to make sure you don't forget any and so that the doctor can address them all. However, when you finally get into her examining room, she rushes you through in less than fifteen minutes, focusing on only one or two issues. You leave wondering, "What happened?"*

*Here's what happened and how to make sure you have enough time in the next visit. It's not the doctor who controls how much time he or she spends with you; it's the scheduler. By using the phrase "follow-up appointment," you inadvertently programmed the scheduler to book ten to fifteen minutes max for you. If you have more than a simple symptom to discuss, bring this up when you make the appointment and let them know that you may need more time. That simple!*

7. Media.

The media plays a significant role in supporting the current culture of care, particularly the "find it and fix it" expectation. Since 1997, when the Food and Drug Administration (FDA) relaxed the rules for direct-to-consumer pharmaceutical advertising (DTCPA),[16] drug manufacturers have increased their ad budgets to capitalize on the estimate that every ad dollar spent increases that drug's sales by $2.20 to $4.20. Since the average American television viewer watches as many as nine drug ads a day, totaling sixteen hours per year, which far exceeds the amount of time the average individual spends with a primary care physician, you can imagine the amount of influence channeled through the media. In addition to DTCPA, since the mid-2000s, television viewers have also been barraged with health news, medical talk shows, medical reality shows, and medical television dramas. The media promotes public health and drives awareness of important medical issues, but they also sensationalize headlines, misrepresent scientific findings, and distort reality in order to provide drama and entertainment. No wonder information-hungry viewers believe in and seek medical miracles and miracle drugs for themselves.

## Facebook Question

*Chopper: I heard your segment on mixed messages the media is sending about whether pregnant women should drink caffeine or not, and the study you cited that showed up to two cups a day doesn't increase the risk of miscarriage or preterm birth. My assistant, who is pregnant, is now avoiding caffeine, deli meat, and a whole slew of other potentially dangerous foods, as she'd read on the Internet. She really misses her latte! Can you send me a link to your segment so I can share it with her?*

*Dr. Georgiou: There is a lot of noise and opinion on the Web, so it's important to stick with evidence-based advice. Here is the link to the recommendations from the American College of Obstetrics and Gynecology regarding caffeine.* [17]

8. Affordable Care Act.

The Affordable Care Act of 2008 has brought several positive results to healthcare access, including making health insurance accessible to 7.2 million more Americans. [18]

The act includes provisions to prevent insurers from denying coverage or charging higher premiums to individuals with preexisting illnesses. Doctors and hospitals will increasingly be paid based on the quality of care they deliver rather than the quantity of care. For consumers, however, the law simply mandates that each person be insured by a comprehensive health insurance policy. There are no provisions in the law that make Americans think twice about the quality of their lifestyle choices. Except for tobacco use, insurers cannot charge higher premiums to individuals with high-risk behaviors such as abusing alcohol, riding a motorcycle without a helmet, or high-risk sexual practices. And there are no provisions that keep consumers accountable for their own health. If a patient has high blood pressure but continues to eat a high salt diet and avoids exercise, his or her doctor prescribes more medication—paid for by insurance, of course. If a patient is readmitted after hip replacement surgery because he or she skipped physical therapy, his or her outcome is damaged by his or her own choices, but he or she is not financially penalized for sabotaging his or her outcome. The hospital and doctor, not the patient, incur the financial penalties for the patient's noncompliance. I believe the ACA reinforces the norm of complacency and, worse, of the patient's passive role in a process that should be collaboration among the doctor, the care team, and, most importantly, the patient . . . or, I should say, consumer.

These eight historical dynamics help explain how we got here. They influence how you interact, how you speak, what you believe, and how you think. These factors have shaped a passive, rule-abiding, quick-fix culture that is holding you back from achieving the quality and quantity of life that you deserve. The important questions to ask are: How do you move forward in a more positive direction? How do you maintain the dynamics that allow you to live in one of the most advanced and prosperous nations in the world while taking the necessary steps to become an advocate for yourself and an active participant in your care?

Behavior is at the core of culture. Changing the culture of care at a national or individual level cannot be regulated or mandated. It must evolve with time, through education and awareness. Change occurs when people feel confident and competent in taking a new approach.

This book is about making a positive change in your approach to your healthcare. I will give you practical examples, checklists, tools, resources, new vocabulary, and other techniques that will help you feel confident and competent in navigating the healthcare system. You will learn to make choices, be a partner in your health, and advocate voraciously for yourself, your family, and other loved ones.

## NOTES

1. KSTP-TV Channel 5, https://www.facebook.com/KSTPTV.

2. Archelle MD, https://www.facebook.com/archellemd. Site was formerly named Create Health with Dr. Archelle Georgiou.

3. Market Research.com, http://www.marketresearch.com/Marketdata-Enterprises-Inc-v416/Weight-Loss-Status-Forecast-8016030/.

4. TECH TIMES, http://www.techtimes.com/articles/28986/20150127/meet-atx-101-new-magic-injection-to-get-rid-of-your-double-chin-yes-no-surgery-needed.htm .

5. "Erectile Dysfunction Drugs Market—Global Industry Analysis, Size, Share, Growth, Trends and Forecast 2013–2019," Transparency Market Research, October 21, 2013, accessed April 16, 2015, https://globenewswire.com/news-release/2015/04/16/725113/10129251/en/Erectile-Dysfunction-Drugs-Market-is-expected-to-reach-an-estimated-value-of-US-3-4-billion-in-2019-Transparency-Market-Research.html.

6. "Prescription Opioid Overdose Data," Centers for Disease Control and Prevention, accessed April 21, 2016, http://www.cdc.gov/drugoverdose/data/overdose.html.

7. "Opioid-Induced Constipation Treatment Market Will Boom to $650M by 2019," *Drug Discovery and Development*, December 2, 2015, accessed April 21, 2016, http://www.dddmag.com/news/2015/12/opioid-induced-constipation-treatment-market-will-boom-650m-2019.

8. America's Health Rankings, United Health Foundation, http://www.americashealthrankings.org/reports/annual#sthash.KDoBQmCr.dpuf.

9. "National Health Expenditure Projections 2012–2022: Forecast Summary," Centers for Medicare and Medicare Services, http://www.cms.gov/Research-Statistics-Data-and-Systems/Statistics-Trends-and-Reports/National-HealthExpendData/downloads/proj2012.pdf.

10. World Values Survey Association, http://www.worldvaluessurvey.org/WVSContents.jsp.

11. Julia Neuberger, "Do We Need a New Word for Patients?" *British Medical Journal* 318 (June 26, 1999): 1756–58, http://dx.doi.org/10.1136/bmj.318.7200.1756.

12. Internal Revenue Code of 1939, Pub. L. No. 1, Sec. 104, 76th Cong. (1939).

13. Internal Revenue Code of 1954, Pub. L. No. 83–591, Sec. 106, 83rd Cong. (1954).

14. "What Americans Don't Know About Their Doctors and Hospital May Be Putting Their Health at Risk," *Healthgrades*, October 23, 2012, http://

www.healthgrades.com/about/press-room/what-americans-dont-know-about-their-doctors-and-hospitals-may-be-putting-their-health-at-risk.

15. Donald K. Cherry, MS, et al., "National Ambulatory Medical Care Survey: 2006 Summary," *National Health Statistics Reports*, no. 3 (August 6, 2008), http://www.cdc.gov/nchs/data/nhsr/nhsr003.pdf.

16. C. Lee Ventola, MS, "Direct-to-Consumer Pharmaceutical Advertising: Therapeutic or Toxic?" *Pharmacy and Therapeutics* 36, no. 10 (October 2011): 669–84, http://www.ncbi.nlm.nih.gov/pmc/articles/PMC3278148/.

17. "No Link Between Moderate Caffeine Consumption and Miscarriage," *The American Congress of Obstetricians and Gynecologists*, July 21, 2010, http://www.acog.org/About-ACOG/News-Room/News-Releases/2010/No-Link-Between-Moderate-Caffeine-Consumption-and-Miscarriage.

18. "ObamaCare Facts: Facts on the Affordable Care Act," Obamacare Facts, accessed April 4, 2016, http://obamacarefacts.com/obamacare-facts/.

# 3

# THE POWER OF PREFERENCES OVER THOUGHT TRAPS

**M**any of the Facebook questions I receive from viewers are simple. But some, like the one from Loise, are about complicated health issues.

Facebook Question

*Loise: I have a three-level cervical spine compression. A laminoplasty was recommended, but now the recommendation has changed to a three-level ACDF (anterior cervical discectomy and fusion). The research tells me the fusion may or may not fuse. I am confused and scared of surgery. Where can I find death stats for this surgery?*

*Dr. Georgiou: Being confused is normal and it's frustrating when you can't get firm answers on the complication rate or the likelihood that the surgery will even relieve the pain. As with all surgeries, there is risk and benefit. While surgery might have complications, not doing anything could also result in complications. The most important issue is to make sure that you are seeing a surgeon who is board certified or fellowship trained in spine surgery in addition to being board certified in neurosurgery or orthopedic surgery.*

I have been moved and concerned about the viewers who resort to writing to me at 10:30 p.m. on a Sunday night about critical health decisions: "Should I have surgery or not? Should I have device A or device B? Or C?" Frequently, these viewers have information overload and do not know how to sort through their options to arrive at the right decision. They are overwhelmed, scared, and simply want someone they *think* they trust to tell them what to do. I can't give my Facebook chatters the definitive direction that they want because I am not their doctor, but I can use my medical knowledge to explain conditions in terms they can understand, lay out options to consider, tee up questions to ask their doctor, and empower them to advocate for themselves.

When a relative or close friend reaches out for help, however, I do have access to the additional information I need, and I transform into an intense patient advocate. This is the email I received from my sister-in-law in March 2015.

> *Hi. I was hoping I wouldn't have to write this, but you probably guessed that something was up. Bottom line is that I was just diagnosed with breast cancer. I have a lumpectomy scheduled next week. Then I'll get radiation. Do you think this is the right decision? I asked my doctor what she would do. She said I could get a mastectomy but she didn't talk a lot about it. I am too emotional to talk so just let me know what you think by email for now. Thanks. Love you.*

Carol is sixty-five years old, healthy, and, except for sitting out in the sun too much, takes good care of herself. She is educated, Web and technology savvy, but was lost in her new diagnosis. Her fear was palpable. The wealth of information on breast cancer felt like too much information. She was drowning in a sea of blood tests, bone scans, biopsies, surgeons, oncologists, radiation therapy, estrogen receptor status, and adjuvant therapy—and didn't know where to start. In one of Carol's follow-up emails, she said, "I just want the doctor to tell me what to do." I gently explained that her doctor's responsibility was to lay out all the options; her responsibility was to decide "what to do."

The first step was for Carol to decide between a modified radical mastectomy and a lumpectomy with radiation. Because her surgeon skimmed over the details, I made sure she understood the pros and cons of each approach. But in order for Carol to make the best decision, I knew she needed one additional test that her doctor had overlooked: BRCA (BReast CAncer) gene testing. While not all women with breast cancer need BRCA testing, Carol is of Ashkenazi Jewish descent, which means her risk of being BRCA positive was 1 in 40 compared to a risk of

1 in 500 in the general population. A credible health information website would have laid out this information for her.

Being BRCA-positive changes the pros and cons of breast cancer treatment options. While lumpectomy plus radiation and mastectomy have similar survival rates in BRCA-negative women, the statistics change in women with a BRCA gene. There is a higher risk of recurrence after lumpectomy and radiation versus mastectomy. In addition, the gene doubles or triples the risk of a second, new breast cancer in the contralateral breast. If Carol were BRCA-positive, a third option would be to have a mastectomy on the affected breast and a prophylactic mastectomy on the healthy breast.

Besides survival and recurrence statistics, Carol worried about the financial aspects of her decision. Would Medicare pay for the BRCA testing? If she chose the mastectomy route, would Medicare cover the prophylactic mastectomy? What about the reconstruction? The answers would impact her decision because she loves going to the beach. If she chose lumpectomy and radiation, what type of radiation would be best—external beam radiation or brachytherapy?

How do you find answers to all of these questions in the midst of a cancer diagnosis? And when you have the answers, how do you sort through them, digest them, and make a decision? Popular media reports that the average American adult makes about 35,000 decisions a day. Many are minor, occur instantaneously, and rarely have long-term consequences: What should I eat for breakfast? Others pave the course for the future: What job offer do I take? Which daycare should I select for my child? You lay out the options, understand the facts, compare risks and benefits, and gather input from experts. Ultimately, however, you know that the final choice can only be made *by you* because it has to be right *for you.*

Most adults say they want to make the decisions that affect their health. That's especially true as the Internet has democratized information—giving everyone access to medical information, drug information, clinical trials, and new research, rather than limiting it to the journals and textbooks published for physicians. In addition, with higher premiums and deductibles, most Americans are paying a higher proportion of their overall healthcare costs. So there is a financial incentive to be a smart consumer of healthcare. In one study, 65 percent of Americans say that *if* they had cancer, they would want to make decisions regarding their care; but only 12 percent of cancer patients actually do.[1] While the majority of people want to be in control of their healthcare decisions, they frequently cede control when they are in the exam room scantily dressed in a blue paper drape.

Why do people abandon the opportunity to participate and retreat to "Doctor, what would you do?" Why do they assume that the doctor has listed *all* the options and blindly trust that the doctor's decision is aligned with what they would have selected if they had all the facts? Because making healthcare decisions is hard. Making serious decisions is even harder and, at a time when people feel most vulnerable, they look for guidance and reassurance. You want to hope that your doctors will make the right decisions for you. However, in healthcare, there is rarely a single option or one right answer, which means doctors apply their personal preferences and biases to arrive at their recommendations. Unfortunately, doctors' and patients' values are not always aligned. In a study of cancer patients, patients' and doctors' decisions were concordant only 38 percent of the time.[2] In the case of breast cancer, patients were significantly less likely than providers to value keeping their breast as a top goal when choosing between lumpectomy and mastectomy surgery—7 percent versus 71 percent.[3] This helps explain the recommendation, and to some extent the sole option, offered by Carol's surgeon. You may be thinking, "But I want my doctor's opinion." Of course you do; you value their expertise and judgment. However, the physician's opinion shouldn't translate into a unilateral decision about your care.

Relinquishing medical decisions to your doctor is not your only decision-making option. Shared decision making (SDM)[4] is a well-known term among healthcare professionals. It is "a process where both patients and physicians share information, express treatment preferences and agree on a treatment plan" based on the fit of the treatment with patient preferences. Studies from as far back as the 1980s show that shared decision making has a positive impact on patients' health.[5] Diabetics[6] who participate in SDM have significantly better control of their blood sugar; individuals with hypertension achieve better blood pressure control; patients with high cholesterol who participate in the decision to take statins (cholesterol lowering drugs) are more diligent[7] about taking their medication regularly. Among patients having open-heart[8] surgery, those who received more information prior to their procedure had less pain and shorter hospital stays.

Ninety-three percent of primary care physicians support SDM principles, but only about 10 percent of healthcare decisions are made using a SDM approach.[9] Physicians frequently complain that there is not enough time during office visits to have conversations with patients about all their options. Many think that patients aren't capable of understanding the scientific evidence. Yet others believe that patients don't want to be involved in decision making and worry that a SDM discussion will diminish the patient's confidence in the physician's expertise.[10]

But it's not all the doctors' fault. People say they are reluctant to initiate or fully engage in shared decision making because they perceive a power imbalance with physicians during interactions. Others don't feel confident asking questions because of their lack of medical knowledge and inability to understand medical jargon.[11] Some just want the doctor to "find it and fix it" and simply aren't willing to invest time and energy in learning about their treatment options and outcomes.[12]

Here is why it's so important to overcome these barriers: doctors and patients bring different expertise to care decisions. Doctors are responsible for evaluating symptoms, establishing the path to a diagnosis, and using evidence-based information to objectively lay out treatment options. Patients are responsible for understanding, identifying, and sharing their unique needs, beliefs, and preferences. Doctors are experts in clinical medicine; patients are experts in themselves. Both are equally important inputs for evaluating risks, benefits, and trade-offs when making healthcare decisions.

Abandoning your responsibility in this process means that instead of getting what you want, your care will be what doctors *think* you want. The reality is that doctors are trained to be experts in diagnosing disease, but they are not trained in diagnosing patients' values. Instead of waiting and hoping for doctors to change the way they practice medicine, this book gives you the tools you need to have a voice about what matters most to you and shows you how to use that voice to get what you need for your health and healthcare.

## PRIORITIES, PREFERENCES, AND PERCEPTIONS

Your personal goals and personality are what make you unique. They are the lens through which you experience the world, shape your perspective, and influence your priorities and preferences. Priorities and preferences both reflect an individual's values, and people frequently use these terms interchangeably, but their definitions are different. A priority is something you think is more important than something else, whereas a preference is something you like more than something else. My priority is eating fruits and vegetables, while my preference is eating salted caramel ice cream.

In healthcare, your priorities and preferences act as guideposts for your choices regarding physical, emotional, and financial well-being. For example:

- Physical: Do you prefer a treatment that restores how your body functions at the expense of how your body looks? Are you more concerned about quality-of-life statistics or duration-of-life statistics?
- Social/Emotional: Are you capable and willing to make a significant lifestyle change to manage your condition or is it more realistic to take daily medication? Do you accept the risk of recurrence (or even death) to stay true to your religious beliefs?
- Financial: Can you afford the financial consequences of a surgery with a long recuperation or do you need a more conservative approach that allows you to continue working?

Priorities and preferences tend to shift based on the circumstances and seriousness of the medical situation. You may not be bothered enough by depression to tolerate the dry mouth and constipation associated with amitriptyline (an antidepressant medication), though you may be willing to tolerate these side effects if you are desperate to get relief from nerve pain, also treated with amitriptyline, after a bout of shingles. Similarly, financial considerations may be important when deciding whether to go to the emergency room for a sore back, but money may be irrelevant if you are facing a life-threatening illness.

Your preferences and priorities do not replace the facts; they complement them. They are subjective and influence your judgment but they are not right or wrong; they are what make you "You." Insight to what's important can help assure that these value-based care decisions are tailored to meet your needs.

Perceptions, on the other hand, can cloud your judgment. Here's why: Humans love order and prefer having explanations for why things happen. So the brain copes with life's randomness by filtering, organizing, and interpreting our experiences so that the world makes more sense. However, these interpretations aren't necessarily fact-based and may be substantially different from reality. Nevertheless, the comfort of these perceptions is so powerful that they can distort the facts and dominate one's thinking.

## Facebook Question

*Patrick: My father is trying to treat my mother's Alzheimer's with mega doses of niacinamide. How can I get him to stop trying "natural" and herbal supplements and listen to medical professionals? He believes any alternative medicine information but doesn't believe doctors because they don't have extensive nutritional training.*

*Dr. Georgiou: This is a tough situation because your father is desperate. The first thing I'd do is give him good information on the known treatments for Alzheimer's. The Alzheimer's Organization is the best I know of. Then, I would make sure that he (and your mother) are going to a doctor who communicates well and listens to them. If your dad feels that the doctor is listening and doing everything possible, he will be less likely to find his own nonscience-based solution.*

Patrick's father is correct that doctors don't have extensive nutritional training, but his perception that "natural" solutions are effective for the treatment of Alzheimer's has no scientific basis. Perceptions are generalizations, assumptions, intuition, or gut instincts that we rely on and believe as truth. I think of them as "thought traps." They speed up the evaluation process and ease the emotional discomfort of complex, chaotic situations, but can lead to wrong decisions and poor health. "Antibiotics always make my cold go away faster." Or "I'm not worried about lung cancer. My father smoked his whole life and was fine." Perceptions, also called biases, are blinders that give us permission to ignore relevant information and narrow our alternatives.[13] For inconsequential situations, these mental short cuts are a low-risk time saver. But when a healthcare situation is serious, they limit objectivity and can be the difference between life and death.

No one is immune from perceptions, but being aware of them can protect you from their negative consequences. Some of the common (mis)perceptions that hijack people's brains when making healthcare decisions are:

- *"My personal risk is lower than average."* Individuals' perception of their personal risk influences their decisions and subsequently their behavior. Smokers underestimate their risk of lung cancer,[14] which reduces the likelihood that they will attempt to quit. My own daughter is misled by her perceptions. She is twenty-four years old and fair skinned with countless moles. She had a biopsy on three moles and the pathology showed "highly atypical" cells. In other words, she is at substantially increased risk for developing melanoma. But she doesn't perceive herself as being at high risk, so she forgets to wear sunscreen and procrastinates scheduling her annual skin exam with the dermatologist. Unfortunately, perceived risk is not actual risk.

- *"I've heard of that."* Familiarity trumps facts. People tend to favor a treatment they have heard of even if they have no real knowledge of that treatment or the alternatives. Familiarity is comfortable and morphs into a perception of "best." Take the example of contraception. Four out of five sexually active women have used oral contraceptives and only 50 percent of women have even heard of an intrauterine device or IUD.[15] As a result "the Pill" (so familiar that it has a nickname) has been the dominant form of female birth control since the 1960s even though IUDs are more effective at preventing pregnancy.[16]

- *"That treatment worked for my friend, my neighbor. . . ."* Past experiences can be a source of wisdom, but they can also be the source of erroneous beliefs and bad decisions. The extreme example is seen in gamblers who tend to overestimate their chances of winning when they believe they are having a lucky streak. In healthcare, people tend to choose a treatment that has worked in the past (for others or for themselves) even if the details of their personal medical situation are different. A patient with a herniated disc is more likely to want surgery (rather than physical therapy and muscle relaxants) if they have a friend whose symptoms were relieved with spine surgery. But if that same friend had a complication or has chronic pain, the patient is likely to be cautious about going under the knife. In either situation, decisions made based on past experiences, and especially the past medical experiences of other individuals, are rolling the dice with your health.

- *"My doctor seems to know what is wrong."* People want to believe and latch on to the first diagnosis they receive about a health issue. This "anchoring bias" offers some certainty. However, having overconfidence in the first opinion creates blinders to other diagnoses and blunts the motivation to seek a second opinion.

- *"I just want to get it done."* People often choose to get care at the local hospital or with the doctor who offers the earliest appointment. While this choice may be a time saver, your brain equates convenience with quality. A survey conducted by Healthgrades showed consumers consider the location of a hospital equally important to the survival and complication rates.[17]

- *"I've done this much. I might as well do this too."* Decisions are influenced by the emotional and financial commitment of previous decisions. Take in vitro fertilization as an example. Studies show that implanting one or two embryos achieves the same pregnancy rate as when three or more embryos are transferred but without the risk of twins or triplets.[18] Having a single fetus decreases the risk of premature birth and mental and physical handicaps. However, because a single IVF cycle can cost between $12,000 and $15,000, prospective parents may lobby their specialist to implant more embryos to get more "bang for the buck."

When facts conflict with perceptions, your brain is a battleground. The reality is that without making an active effort to stay objective, the natural tendency is to give in to your perceptions. They are a quick route to your comfort zone. In medicine, if your perceptions win the battle, your health may lose the war. A famous example that illustrates this point is Steve Jobs's approach to managing his pancreatic cancer. When Jobs was diagnosed in 2003, his early treatment choices were unconventional. He rejected potentially life-saving surgery in favor of alternative treatments like herbs and carrot juice. Walter Isaacson,

Jobs's biographer, described him as having a "reality distortion field." In an interview with ABC, Isaacson said, "I just think that he has such belief in his power of magical thinking that, in this case, it failed him." Ultimately, Steve Jobs regretted the early decisions he made about his care, but by that point, it was too late.[19]

How do you remain objective about your diagnosis and treatment options and stay true to your preferences while recognizing and rejecting perceptions that distort your decision making? How do you make choices that result in satisfaction rather than regret? Feeling good about your decision is influenced by the outcome and by *how* you made the decision. Studies show that people feel remorse about a decision when they realize they could have made a better choice by looking at more information and weighing the pros and cons carefully.[20]

The approach I use when making my own healthcare choices and helping others with theirs is not based on information I found in medical textbooks, but rather in ethics textbooks. Ethical dilemmas, like medical ones, are complex. They require individual context and rarely have one right answer. Ethical decision-making tools help us focus on all the relevant dimensions of what are usually very personal health issues.

I was first introduced to ethical decision-making tools for healthcare issues in 1994 when I was at CIGNA. My job, as one of CIGNA's medical directors, was to stamp "approve" or "deny" when patients needed healthcare services. The majority of these requests were routine insurance determinations. On occasion, however, there were complex, sometimes tragic, situations that did not fit neatly into the contractual language or medical necessity guidelines that we used to make our decisions.

CIGNA recognized that we were struggling with ethical dilemmas; there were no right or wrong answers, yet we were obligated to make a decision about whether or not we would pay for an individual's requested medical care. CIGNA invited Dr. Arthur Caplan, an internationally known medical ethicist from the University of Pennsylvania, to show us how to use ethical decision-making tools in these healthcare situations.

I don't recall the specific details of the many cases we evaluated with Caplan's tools, but I do remember feeling at peace with the decisions because our new approach to these heart-wrenching, difficult situations was holistic and thoughtful. While the process Caplan introduced may sound simplistic, his systematic approach guided us to

- gather the facts,
- formulate the alternatives, and
- weigh the pros and cons

*before* making a final decision. These steps kept us from taking mental shortcuts and falling into our own perception thought traps. Initially, we kept laminated cards on our desks to remind us of the step-by-step approach we needed to follow. Over time, this method became second nature and I found myself applying it to more routine decisions. In the years since I left CIGNA, I've tailored the basic concepts of ethical decision making into what I call the CARES model. I use the model for personal healthcare decisions, to help friends and relatives who call for advice and to guide viewers who ask me questions.

The rest of this chapter explains the CARES model. Using this model, you can become actively involved in your care and make choices that are aligned with your priorities and preferences. Even if you are not faced with an illness or medical issue right now, learning and using the CARES approach can help you to develop confidence that you can make the right healthcare choices. I want this tool to keep you from feeling lost if a doctor says, "I have bad news."

## CARES MODEL

The CARES model includes five key steps:

- Understand Your **Condition**.
- Know Your **Alternatives**.
- **Respect** Your Preferences.
- **Evaluate** Your Options.
- **Start** Taking Action.

## Step 1: Understand Your Condition

The CARES model, and the decision-making process, begins with understanding your medical condition. This may seem obvious because most people can cite their diagnosis and recognize their own symptoms. However, studies show that patients often overestimate what they really know about their disease. In a study of patients needing a bone marrow transplant, 77 percent thought they had enough information, but when asked specific questions, only about 52 percent demonstrated knowledge of the facts.[21] Similarly, a study of diabetic patients showed that even among those who had attended a training program, almost half didn't understand how to properly care for themselves.[22] Understanding your condition means being able to answer "so what?"

Facebook Question

*Bob: My blood pressure is 160/95. Do I need to treat my blood pressure with medication?*

Bob's blood pressure is merely a measurement. "So what?" A healthy blood pressure measurement does not exceed 120/80. If you were able to look inside Bob's body, you would see that his heart is using higher than normal force to push blood into the body's arteries because the resistance in the blood vessels is high. "So what?" High blood pressure is like a continuous mini-workout for the heart. In order to get good circulation, Bob's heart muscle adds about three quarters of a pound of pressure to every heartbeat—twenty-four hours a day, seven days a week. "So what?" Over time, the heart muscle gets fatigued and eventually becomes so weak that it is unable to pump enough blood to the rest of the body. The risk: heart failure. Thirty percent of the U.S. population has high blood pressure, but only about 50 percent are adequately treated. I suspect this dreadful statistic would improve if more people understood the "so what?" of their blood pressure measurement.

Make sure you understand the "so what?" of any number, measurement, laboratory value, x-ray result, or multisyllabic medical diagnosis. Make sure you know why it matters. Getting to the answers may require some research and reading, but it does not require going to medical school or having a clinician's depth of knowledge. It means collecting enough knowledge about the risks (or the lack of risks) of your situation so that you can make informed choices about your treatment options.

## Step 2: Know Your Alternatives

For many conditions, there are an array of treatment approaches that can include lifestyle changes, medication, radiation, surgery, or simply watching and doing nothing. The details of your clinical condition will dictate the treatment options available to you. Patients with cardiovascular disease and blockage in multiple arteries, for example, can either undergo traditional open-heart surgery, minimally invasive heart surgery (an approach that avoids stopping the heart), or stent placements. For women who have uterine fibroid tumors, there are three different surgical approaches a gynecologist can use to perform a hysterectomy. In some situations, the hysterectomy can be avoided completely by having a radiologist inject clotting medication into the fibroid's blood vessels to cut off blood flow and shrink the tumor.

Facebook Question

*Stevie: I am trying my third month of a CPAP machine. I can't stand wearing it: I feel suffocated and strangled. I think that they (the docs) are going to kick me off of it because Medicare won't pay for it if I don't use it all the time. Can you suggest an alternative?*

*Dr. Georgiou: Some people with mild to moderate sleep apnea can be treated with a dental device that is much more comfortable than using a CPAP machine. The device looks like a retainer, and it works by moving the jaw forward and opening the airway. Because these are prescribed by dentists, most medical doctors aren't familiar with oral appliances as an alternative to CPAP. You should talk to your doctor and then get evaluated by a dentist who specializes in sleep apnea.*

People expect that doctors objectively lay out all the options for their care. Only 20 percent of people raise the topic of a new treatment option with their provider.[23] Unfortunately, just as you have biases, physicians also have biases that can lead them to recommend one treatment over another, even if there are alternative treatments offering the same or even better outcomes. Everyone has a tendency to feel more comfortable with approaches that are familiar. Medical specialists in particular tend to focus on treatments that are within the scope of their own training and specialty. In some cases, this can lead physicians to completely exclude valid options from the conversation. For example, when a cancer patient has nausea related to chemotherapy, oncologists routinely prescribe medications called 5-HT3 antagonists, such as Zofran and Kytril. However, acupuncture is also an option that should be considered because studies have shown that it too can relieve nausea and vomiting symptoms. In the CARES model, "knowing your alternatives" means being aware of all the treatment options for your particular situation that are backed by scientific evidence verifying effectiveness. This includes complementary and alternative medicine (CAM) treatments when there is reasonable proof that they have some effectiveness for a particular condition or symptoms.

How do you find out about feasible alternatives that aren't mentioned by your doctor? Knowing your alternatives means asking your doctor, "What else?"

- Are 100 percent of the patients with this condition treated one way?
- What other treatments are available in addition to what you have recommended?
- What are the pros and cons of each alternative?
- Is there anything I can do to self-manage this condition?

## Step 3: Respect Your Preferences

In hypothetical situations, only 9 percent of Americans want their doctor to make healthcare choices on their behalf. Sixty-two percent say that they prefer to participate in their healthcare decisions and deliberate with their physician about their treatment options.[24] However, when you are facing an illness, you feel vulnerable, scared, and overwhelmed. Your feelings have an impact on your approach to your care. Your tendency is to ask your doctor, "What would you do?" While the question is reasonable, too often people simply defer to the doctor's judgment to determine their treatment plan.

Here's the problem with relying on the physician as the sole decision maker: physicians are human too (yes, that is a fact). Without knowing your personal preferences, they use their personal lens—their cultural background, religious and cultural beliefs, and local norms—to judge risks versus benefits, harm versus safety, and the consequences of treatment on your quality of life. Doctors, like all people, bring their own perceptions, biases, and blinders to their recommendations. To complicate this further, what doctors recommend to patients is different from what they recommend for themselves. One study showed that 38 percent of doctors selected a higher-risk treatment for colon cancer for themselves, but only 25 percent recommended this treatment to patients. When surveyed about a high-risk treatment for avian flu, the majority of physicians did not choose to get immunized themselves but tended to recommend immunizations for their patients.[25]

Whether doctors should even make recommendations to their patients is controversial. Some experts feel that doctors should simply lay out the options and let patients decide what to do. Others believe that physicians should help patients make informed choices by using their medical knowledge and experience to make recommendations. The common area of agreement, however, is that only a patient can decide whether the risks and side effects of a particular treatment are worth the opportunity for symptom relief and a cure. Most importantly, when patients are actively involved in the decision, it increases the likelihood that they will adhere to the plan and ultimately benefit from treatment.[26]

## Facebook Question

*Gale: I have Afib and I will NOT take blood thinners due to side effects. I choose to just take half an aspirin a day. Am I being foolish?*

*Dr. Georgiou: I can tell you the facts and then you can weigh the risks and benefits and make a decision based on your priorities. With Afib, you have a five-times higher risk of stroke. Your annual risk is 2.5 to 4 percent. The risk gets higher as you age. Anticoagulants reduce the risk of a first stroke in Afib patients by 68 percent. While aspirin decreases the risk a bit, it is not as effective as anticoagulants (blood thinners).*

Gale's adamancy ("I will NOT take blood thinners) seemed to contradict her question ("Am I foolish?"). The bleeding risks associated with anticoagulants are lower than the devastating stroke risks associated with untreated atrial fibrillation (an irregular heart rhythm). As a physician, I encourage patients with this condition to take blood thinners unless there is a major contraindication. However, the risk that Gale was willing to take is her decision, not mine.

When you are evaluating healthcare options, the key to identifying preferences is asking yourself, "What matters most?" The question itself can feel overwhelming, but preferences typically fit into four major categories:

- Medical preferences: Chance of a cure or recovery versus the risk of complications or death; recovery time. How much medical risk are you willing to take to improve your health?
- Quality of life: Level and duration of pain; dependence on others; need for long-term monitoring or medication. How willing are you to tolerate short-term and long-term restrictions that affect your quality of life?
- Financial preferences: Costs covered by insurance versus out-of-pocket expenses; time away from work, school, or family responsibilities. How much of a financial commitment are you willing or able to make to achieve your health goal?
- Personal: Cultural and religious beliefs; fears; convenience; other sociocultural factors.

### Step 4: Evaluate Your Options

Understanding your condition, knowing your options, and acknowledging your preferences gives you the information to confidently move to Step 4, evaluating your options and making a decision.

As you deliberate, the question that can help guide you to the right decision is: What gives me peace of mind—now and for the future?

- Which treatment options address the concerns that are your priorities?
- Which treatment options have acceptable short- and long-term risks?

- Which decision has quality-of-life trade-offs that you can defend to yourself and the people who love you?
- Which treatments have an acceptable financial responsibility?
- Which decision lets you sleep at night knowing that you made the right choice for you?
- Which decision will keep you from feeling regret?

Choosing between options is the most difficult step in the CARES model. All too frequently, none of the options is a clear front-runner. Because there is no right or wrong answer, you assume some responsibility, and the stakes can be high. Yes, it is scary to weigh in on whether to choose high-dose chemotherapy versus a bone marrow transplant for a life-threatening acute leukemia. It is also handwringing to decide whether the miscarriage risk associated with an amniocentesis outweighs the benefit of genetic information obtained from the test. For complex situations, these decisions are best made with a physician. However, instead of being a passive listener, you can use Steps 1 through 3 to gather the information you need to have an intelligent—bidirectional and nonhierarchical—conversation with your doctor.

In this "shared decision making" interaction, you and the physician spend an equal amount of time talking and listening because both of you bring equally important points of view to the discussion. But only you can make the decision that is in harmony with your life and lifestyle. Only you know the decision that gives you peace and makes it easy for you to sleep at night. Regardless of the outcome, studies show that when patients are well informed about their options and participate in the process, expectations are more realistic[27] and there is less regret even if there is a less than ideal outcome.

## Step 5: Start Taking Action

Being a partner in your care is an ongoing process. It starts with making or participating in healthcare decisions and continues as you take responsibility for the medications, appointments, tests, procedures, monitoring, and lifestyle changes that translate decisions into actions. As U.S. surgeon general C. Everett Koop said, "Drugs don't work in patients who don't take them." On average, only 50 percent of people take their medications as prescribed; this statistic holds even among people with chronic illness. There are many underlying reasons for nonadherence, but some of the common ones are forgetfulness, perceived side effects, cost issues, and a belief that the medication isn't really necessary. [28]

A common coping mechanism is to "take one day at a time" so that you focus on dealing with today and not worrying about the future. This mindset can relieve some short-term anxiety but, once again, reinforces a passive relationship with the physician and fuels a lack of accountability to the care plan. Alternatively, when you understand your treatment roadmap (your role, the process, and the reasons), you are empowered to communicate with your physician, ask the *right* questions, and be assertive about your needs.

To follow through on your decisions and to continue making the right choices for your care, you have to take action and ask, "What next?"

- What (exactly) do you have to do over the next thirty, sixty, ninety days? How will your life—work, activities, energy, sex, driving—be different? If there is an aspect of the regimen that isn't compatible with your life and lifestyle, you have to speak up and negotiate a more compatible approach.
- What side effects can you expect? Understand when bumps in the road can be safely addressed at home and when they are serious enough to require medical attention. Anticipating complications may feel scary, but preparation arms you with information that can prevent overreacting, getting discouraged, and feeling tethered to a 24/7 lifeline with your physician.
- What are the indicators that show that this treatment plan is working or not working? You must have the courage to discuss "what's next" if your health is not progressing as you expected. Know when it is time to reconsider options and change course.

The remaining chapters of this book will dive into more detail about the five steps of the CARES model and provide specific "how to" recommendations for accomplishing each of the steps. The examples in this chapter and chapters 4 through 6 highlight how the model can be used to make decisions in the face of a serious illness, including how to integrate complementary and alternative approaches and how to approach aging and end-of-life decisions. However, the CARES model isn't limited to medical decisions. With a few modifications, this model can be used to make other important choices that have an impact on healthcare: chapters 7 and 8 will explain how to use CARES to make the best choice when selecting physicians and buying health insurance. In chapter 9, I will show you how the model can be used to make minor decisions that don't require the input or advice of a physician or care professional at all. Chapter 10 consolidates the CARES model tools laid out in the book. Once you understand how to use the CARES approach, you can refer back to this final chapter as a quick reference guide when you are facing a healthcare decision.

No skill is acquired overnight, and it takes time to assimilate new knowledge. As we move through the CARES approach together, you will be acquiring tools that will empower you to make better health care decisions that align with your priorities, preferences, and personal goals.

## NOTES

1. Barry Schwartz, *Paradox of Choice* (New York: HarperCollins, 2007), 32, accessed April 14, 2016, http://wp.vcu.edu/univ200choice/wp-content/uploads/sites/5337/2015/01/The-Paradox-of-Choice-Barry-Schwartz.pdf.

2. E. Bruera, "Patient Preferences Versus Physician Perception of Treatment Decisions in Cancer Care," *Journal of Clinical Oncology* 19, no. 11 (June 1, 2001).

3. C. N. Lee et al., "Development of Instruments to Measure the Quality of Breast Cancer Treatment Decisions," *Health Expectations* 13, no. 3 (2010).

4. M. E. Peek et al., "Barriers and Facilitators to Shared Decision Making Among African-Americans with Diabetes," *Journal of General Internal Medicine* 24, no. 10 (2009): 1135–39.

5. Cathy Charles et al., "Shared Decision-Making in the Medical Encounter: What Does It Mean? (Or It Takes At Least Two to Tango)," *Social Science and Medicine* 44, no. 5 (1997): 681–92, http://emed.einstein.yu.edu/auth/pdf/138898.pdf.

6. Sheldon Greenfield et al., "Patients' Participation in Medical Care," *Journal of General Internal Medicine* 3, no. 5 (1988): 448.

7. A. J. Weymiller et al., "Helping Patients with Type 2 Diabetes Mellitus Make Treatment Decisions: Statin Choice Randomized Trial," *Archives of Internal Medicine* 167, no. 10 (2007): 1076–82.

8. Heike I. M. Mahler and James A. Kulik, "Preferences for Health Care Involvement, Perceived Control and Surgical Recovery: A Prospective Study," *Social Science and Medicine* 31, no. 7 (1990): 743–51.

9. Clarence H. Braddock et al., "Informed Decision Making in Outpatient Practice: Time to Get Back to Basics," *Journal of the American Medical Association* 282, no. 24 (December 22, 1999): 2313–20, doi:10.1001/jama.282.24.2313.

10. *Informing and Involving Patients in Medical Decisions: The Primary Care Physicians' Perspective* (Informed Medical Decisions Foundation, February 2009), http://informedmedicaldecisions.org/wp-content/uploads/2009/02/PCP_Perspective_WhitePaper.pdf.

11. Peek et al., "Barriers and Facilitators to Shared Decision Making Among African-Americans with Diabetes."

12. Albert G. Mulley et al., *Patients' Preferences Matter: Stop the Silent Diagnosis* (London: The King's Fund, 2012).

13. California Health Care Foundation Article (2005).

14. N. D. Weinstein, "Smokers' Unrealistic Optimism About Their Risk," *Tobacco Control* 14, no. 1 (February 2005): 55–59.

15. Alexandra Sifferlin, "Why Is the Most Effective Form of Birth Control—the IUD—Also the One No One Is Using?" *Time*, June 30, 2014, http://time.com/the-best-form-of-birth-control-is-the-one-no-one-is-using/.

16. K. Daniels et al., "Contraceptive Methods Women Have Ever Used: United States, 1982–2010," *National Health Statistics Reports* 62 (February 14, 2013).

17. "What Americans Don't Know About Their Doctors and Hospital May Be Putting Their Health at Risk," *Healthgrades*, October 23, 2012, http://www.healthgrades.com/about/press-room/what-americans-dont-know-about-their-doctors-and-hospitals-may-be-putting-their-health-at-risk.

18. D. A. Lawlor and S. M. Nelson, "Effect of Age on Decisions about the Numbers of Embryos to Transfer in Assisted Conception: A Prospective Study," *The Lancet* 379 (2012): 521.

19. "Steve Jobs Biographer Walter Isaacson on the Apple CEO's Polarizing Persona," interview by Ned Potter, ABC News, October 23, 2011, accessed August 21, 2015, http://abcnews.go.com/Technology/steve-jobs-biographer-walter-isaacson-apple-ceos-polarizing/story?id=14789445.

20. A. Sagi and N. Friedland, "The Cost of Richness: The Effect of the Size and Diversity of Decision Sets on Post-Decision Regret," *Journal of Personality and Social Psychology* 93, no. 4 (2007).

21. P. J. Stiff et al., "Patients' Understanding of Disease Status and Treatment Plan at Initial Hematopoietic Stem Cell Transplantation Consultation," *Bone Marrow Transplantation* 37, no. 5 (2006): 479–84.

22. Leona Miller et al., "Evaluation of Patients' Knowledge of Diabetes Self-Care," *Diabetes Care* 1, no. 5 (September/October 1978): 275–80.

23. "From Hope to Cures: PhRMA's Second Annual Health Survey" (key findings from a nationwide survey among 1,207 adults conducted June 30–July 6, 2014), http://www.phrma.org/sites/default/files/pdf/Second-Annual-PhRMA-Health-Short.pdf.

24. Elizabeth Murray et al., "Clinical Decision-Making: Patients' Preferences and Experiences," *Patient Education and Counseling* 65, no. 2 (February 2007): 189–96.

25. Peter A. Ubel, MD, et al., "Physicians Recommend Different Treatments for Patients than They Would Choose for Themselves," *Archives of Internal Medicine, JAMA Internal Medicine* 3171, no. 7 (April 11, 2011): 630–34.

26. M. Holmes-Rovner et al., "Patient Satisfaction with Health Care Decisions: The Satisfaction with Decision Scale," *Medical Decision Making* 16, no. 1 (January–March 1996): 56–64.

27. Dawn Stacey et al., "Decision Aids for People Facing Health Treatment or Screening Decisions," *Cochrane Database of Systematic Reviews* 1 (2014), doi: 10.1002/14651858.CD001421.pub4.

28. "Patient Nonadherence: Tools for Combating Persistence and Compliance Issues," *Frost and Sullivan* (December 2005), accessed September 21, 2015, www.frost.com/prod/servlet/cpo/115071625.pdfý.

# 4

# BRING PERSONAL PRIORITIES TO MEDICAL CARE

**F**acebook Question

*Gerry: What are the treatments for hyatal herneia of the stomach?*

*Dr. Georgiou: When someone has a hiatal hernia, the treatment focuses on decreasing the amount of acid reflux—stomach acid that splashes into the esophagus—that causes heartburn symptoms. The most common treatments are anti-acid medications such as H2-blockers (like Zantac®) or proton pump inhibitors (like Prilosec®). A home remedy that can also help is sleeping on a few firm pillows instead of laying flat. When the chest is elevated above the stomach, gravity keeps the acid in the stomach where it belongs. Depending on the severity of the symptoms, surgery may be considered though this is not particularly common.*

Gerry's misspelling of his diagnosis was a clue that he wasn't very familiar with the details of his condition, yet he wanted to jump to the treatment. My response told him what he wanted to know but also what he needed to know—the "so what?" of hiatal hernia. The basic information I shared about acid reflux explained why and how anti-acid medications work, and the quick anatomy lesson explained how some minor lifestyle modifications might decrease his symptoms. In a few sentences, I armed him with some facts he could use to participate in his own care.

If I had more time, I would have gone into more detail. The acid splashes into the esophagus because the valve between the esophagus and stomach becomes overly relaxed or weak. Obesity puts physical pressure on the abdomen, further weakens the valve's function, and makes the symptoms worse. Alcohol and cigarettes, along with spicy foods and caffeine, can trigger opening of the valve as well. Besides discomfort, the more important "so what?" of reflux is the long-term risk. Having chronic symptoms can cause tissue inflammation that can lead to scar tissue, narrowing of the esophagus, esophageal ulcers, or even precancerous changes. For Gerry, more information would help him decide whether to get an endoscopy now versus waiting to see if his symptoms resolve with medication. Both are reasonable options. The CARES model hinges on being knowledgeable about your condition, but the benefits go well beyond decision making.

All too often, physicians state a diagnosis and the recommended treatment with a level of finality and brevity that doesn't invite questions or clarifications. They dual-task, talking to patients while simultaneously entering information into the electronic medical record, and the medical jargon is intimidating. This scenario is not one that makes it comfortable to ask questions about the prescriptions, follow-up tests, procedures, therapy, and medical devices. Most people need motivation to undertake treatment that can be uncomfortable, inconvenient, or expensive. Without some rationale, why bother? If you don't understand why it's important to do something, it's unlikely that you'll be motivated to do it. Think back to being a child. Your mom or dad may have told you to clean up your room . . . "or else." If you asked "why?" they may have responded with "Because I said so." Psychologists believe that this interaction feels insulting to children's intelligence, damages their self-esteem, and makes them feel insignificant and powerless. And when the "or else" threats are vague and poorly defined, the resulting behavior is defiance.

This dynamic also occurs in the exam room. "Take this medication." "Get this MRI." "You need to stop drinking." Physicians (hopefully) don't intentionally make these unilateral statements of authority. Nevertheless, the consequence of paternalistic posture and off-putting communication is the same. There is no "why." The subliminal message from physicians is "Because I said so," and patients don't feel empowered to ask questions. What happens next? They passively nod in agreement, feeling subconscious defiance, and then don't follow the treatment plan. In the United States, nonadherence is estimated to cause approximately 125,000 deaths and at least 10 percent of hospitalizations. Patient defiance costs the U.S. healthcare system between $100 billion and $289 billion annually.[1]

## Facebook Question

*Valerie: What is an ulcer on your ankle area caused from and why is it taking more than five months for it to go away?*

*Dr. Georgiou: Venous skin ulcers are open wounds that usually form on the lower leg when the leg veins don't keep the blood moving back toward the heart. Even after an ulcer heals, new venous ulcers can develop, especially in people who don't use compression stockings, the gold standard for both prevention and treatment.*

Valerie was asking a very basic question despite having a nonhealing ulcer for five months. I wasn't optimistic that she was taking the necessary step her condition requires: wearing compression stockings to care for the ulcer on her ankle. Studies show that 90 percent of patients with this condition purchase the stockings, but less than 60 percent wear them[2] consistently for even a month, and 22 percent don't wear them at all.[3] Because compression stockings are not particularly attractive or comfortable to wear, it's not surprising that patients who are most likely to toss them aside are those who are unfamiliar with the pathophysiology of venous ulcers and don't understand why and how compression stockings work. Being knowledgeable, on the other hand, makes it easier to push through treatment obstacles. Good information provides the rationale to make yourself and your care a priority. For a patient with venous stasis ulcers, this means that despite the fact that compression stockings are thick, warm, and tight, their advantages outweigh their disadvantages.

Many chronic illnesses progress slowly with very subtle symptoms. When people don't understand the "so what?" it can prevent delays in care. If Gerry's reflux causes scarring and mild narrowing of his esophagus, he may not have overt symptoms early on because he naturally accommodates by cutting food into smaller, easier-to-swallow pieces. Knowing the potential complications, however, makes him apt to notice the minor change in his eating habits and could prompt him to call his doctor rather than waiting until he has a full-blown obstruction with a chunk of steak lodged in his esophagus.

Gerry is also more likely to call his doctor ASAP if he has worsening "heartburn" symptoms when he is walking or taking a flight of steps rather than when lying down. Understanding his condition means recognizing that the same symptoms with a different symptom *pattern* might not be reflux at all but rather the early warning sign of a heart attack. Similarly, someone with mild congestive heart failure may feel more short of breath. Is it worsening of their heart condition or pneumonia? Someone with rheumatoid arthritis notices new knee pain. Is it progression of their autoimmune disease (RA) or run of the mill "wear and tear" arthritis that develops with age?

In each situation, you make a decision about whether a symptom is routine, urgent, or emergent and whether you can handle a problem on your own or need professional care. Like it or not, you function as the self-manager of your health.

Comprehending basic anatomy and the details of a disease process is well within the grasp of an average layperson. Yet for many, the inner workings of the human body are a mystery. Research studies showed that only about 50 percent of the general public can accurately identify the location of body organs, and the results were no better among patients with organ-specific[4] disease. A smaller percentage know basic physiology, how each organ functions, and how the body's eleven distinct organ systems work together to make you whole. Without an appreciation of the body's moving parts, your ability to manage your care is severely hampered. When you don't understand, why should you bother?

Given the opportunity, people do want to know what is allowing them to be walking, talking, breathing, thinking human beings. Since 2003, forty million people[5] around the world have visited the Body Worlds exhibitions. Using an odorless preservation process called plastination rather than formaldehyde, these exhibitions put human bodies, organ systems, individual organs, and tissue slices on display. Body Worlds was the first exhibit in which the general public could see a nonsuperficial view of themselves in a healthy and unhealthy state with the "so what?" of diseases and destructive lifestyle choices on full display. A study of visitor reactions not only showed that 86 percent felt better informed about the anatomy of the human body; 43 percent were motivated to pursue a healthier lifestyle.[6] When you are well informed, you are more likely to have a high sense of self-efficacy—confidence that you are capable of self-managing your healthcare. The mindset is "I think I can, so I will—and I'll keep trying—because it's important."

So how do you get there? While many snicker at getting information from "Dr. Google," the explosive access to health information on the Internet is what makes it possible for consumers to be active participants in their health. Yes, it has pitfalls. Anyone with an opinion, from professionals to marketers to indiscriminate bloggers, can publish information. Vulnerable readers who pursue the wrong Internet trail can be misled by inaccurate information and suffer needless anxiety about diseases. The key is knowing what questions you are trying to answer, how and where to find those answers, what to believe, what to ignore, and when to stop searching because you are well-enough informed.

The most common approach that people take when using the Web for health information is to use a search engine such as Google or Yahoo. If the search words are limited to the name of the condition (for example, "diabetes" or "heart attack"), then the top search results will almost always include one or two reliable health information sites, but they may also include sites that have a hidden bias. For example, Google's top search results for "arthritis" include WebMD.com as well as arthritis.org and arthritis.com. The .org is an advocacy organization and their website offers good, comprehensive information. However, the .com website has a heavy focus on medication treatment options, probably because it is owned and supported by a pharmaceutical company that makes arthritis medications.

Not all pharmaceutical sites are biased; not all nonprofit advocacy sites are balanced. Research tells us that only 39 percent of top sites[7] searched give correct health information, so you need to be the arbiter of credibility for each and every site that you access. Unfortunately, people judge the credibility of a site based on initial perceptions—design, typography, font size, and color schemes, rather than its content.[8] And unfortunately, the sites with the most credible sources of information—academic institutions, medical journals, and research-driven nonprofit health advocacy organizations—are least likely to care about or have the funds to prioritize and invest in their site aesthetics.

My recommendation: resist the temptation to do a Google-type search. Instead (and in advance of having your next health crisis or question), take the time to identify one favorite "go to" health information site that you bookmark and use as the starting point for your search. The site I use consistently is MayoClinic.org because it has a clear, predictable layout across all their health topics. After a few repeat visits, it is easy to know the sections or tabs with the information you need to answer your questions. When I want some additional multimedia tools like photographs and videos, I use WebMD.com. Both sites have credible content on a broad range of topics. They are updated regularly and have the requisite HON (Health On the Net) certified badge, a recognized standard regarding the quality of online health information.

## CARES MODEL

### Steps 1 and 2: Understand Your Condition and Know Your Alternatives

I have found that MayoClinic.org is a "one stop shop." For the vast majority of conditions, it is comprehensive enough to fully address the questions you need to ask in order to Understand Your Condition and Know Your Alternatives. Each topic is typically organized into pages that parallel how doctors think and how you *should* think. Each section begins with an explanation of the condition, symptoms, causes, risk factors, and complications—the "so what?"—and conventional treatments, alternative/complementary treatments, and prognosis—the "what else?" Whether you are getting information about your condition from your physician or the Internet, the sequence of questions is the same.

For Step 1 of the CARES model, get smart about your condition. Focus on answering "so what?" and "why bother?"

- What is this condition? If you were able look inside your body, what would you see and how is that different from what you would see if your body was functioning normally?

- What causes this condition? Is it inherited or genetic? Is it infectious? How is it affected by lifestyle choices?
- What is the risk? Does this condition threaten your health? How? Is it reversible? When should this condition be treated to avoid worsening symptoms and greater risk to your health?
- Is it urgent? Emergent? Is it a chronic condition? Does it need treatment or will it resolve on its own?

For Step 2 of the CARES model, focus on answering "what else?"

- Are 100 percent of people with this condition treated one way? (The answer will be "no.") What are the circumstances that make other options available? How does your clinical condition affect your options?
- What other treatments are available in addition to what's been recommended? If you don't want to have the surgery (have the test, take this medication, etc.), what other alternatives are there?
- What else can you do? What are the pros and cons of each alternative?
- Is there anything you can do to self-manage this condition?

Stay focused on finding the answers to these questions. Avoid meandering through a maze of other distracting information. And once you find the sections you need within the site, read them and write (or type) the answers in your own words. The average page visit on the Web lasts a little less than a minute and users only read about one-quarter of the text,[9] but there is no shortcut to spending the time it takes to translate information into the knowledge you need to participate in making decisions about your health.

### Archelle's Insider Tip

*One of the many benefits of doing a regular healthy segment on television is that it forces me to learn about a new health topic well enough to explain it to viewers. How do you know if you really have a grasp on your health condition and the treatment alternatives? Challenge yourself to explain your condition as well as the causes, risk factors, potential complications, and treatment options to a spouse or a friend. If you have read about your health issue and really learned it, then you should be able to teach it in about four minutes, which is the length of each of my segments. In summary: read it, learn it, teach it.*

On occasion, a health information site does not include the most current research discoveries and treatment options that may be available. And your doctor may not mention them either because there is not enough evidence to recommend them or because your doctor simply may not be aware of the new information. Doctors are responsible for their own continuing education and may not have seen information about a medical advance or new treatment. For serious life-threatening conditions and even for conditions requiring surgery or an implantable device, you deserve to be aware of all the options, even those that are still in the experimental phase and not yet proven to be as effective as mainstream treatments. While you may still choose conventional treatment, being thorough in your research will minimize the risk that you might regret your decision in the future.

There is not one "go to" source or website to find the latest research, drug, and technology developments for all conditions. Instead, physicians usually read "review articles" to refresh themselves and update what they need to know about a particular topic. These articles do not reveal new science; rather, they synthesize other credible published data. You can find them by using a general search engine to type in the condition name followed by "review article." Identifying the best article takes a bit of trial and error. I recommend looking for articles that have been either been published in a medical journal within the last three years *or* published on a .gov site. These are the most reliable and well-vetted sources.

Archelle's Insider Tip

*A caution about relying on unpublished articles on .edu sites: While these articles are published by universities or medical institutions, they are usually written to promote the specialists and advanced care treatments offered by their institution. The potential for bias makes these articles a less reliable source of credible information.*

Exploring all the options was helpful to our own family when my mother-in-law, Faye, needed to have valve replacement surgery for aortic stenosis. Faye was a young ninety years old. With the exception of shortness of breath that limited her ability to walk, she was completely healthy. She lived independently in Florida, played mahjong twice a week, and went out for dinner—the early bird of course—with her girlfriends on Fridays. Despite the fact that she didn't look a day older than seventy, we knew that her age made having open heart surgery a significant risk. David and I had heard that some surgeons were doing aortic valve replacements using a transfemoral approach that threads the valve through the artery in the leg instead of opening the chest. The major advantage would be less postoperative pain because the ribs and chest muscles wouldn't have to heal. The disadvantage, based on the scant data available, was a higher risk of stroke. We opted for the open-heart approach and Faye sailed through the surgery and was chatting with me a few hours after leaving the recovery room. Unfortunately, on the night before she was discharged, Faye passed away. A small artery located close to the valve was nicked during the surgery—but no one noticed. Three days later she bled to death. Unfortunate? Tragic. Regret that we didn't guide her toward a surgeon performing the other procedure? None. Faye's biggest fear wasn't death. It was having and surviving a debilitating stroke. Studies published within a year after Faye died showed that the transfemoral procedure would have been safer. Nevertheless, we didn't look back. We were comfortable that we helped Faye make the best decision based on her personal preferences and the data we had at the time.

To complete Step 2, you need to understand the implication of your alternatives. Think about the last time you made a big purchase: a car, a house, a large appliance. Mired in all the details, you likely grabbed a piece of paper, drew a line down the middle, selected key categories (for example, cost, performance, warranty), and listed the pros and cons in bullet points. Use that same process to compare your healthcare choices. Create a chart and list all the options, including "do nothing," in the top row. (Reminder: not taking action also has risks and benefits that are important to recognize and consider.) Then list the categories below in the first column. Tease through your "go to" site and fill in the information on:

- Short-term benefits and advantages: how quickly the treatment works.

- Short-term harms, risks, disadvantages: expected pain, recovery time, or disability; potential complications or side effects.
- Long-term benefits and advantages: likelihood of treatment effectiveness; chance of a cure or survival.
- Long-term harms, risks, disadvantages: risk of recurrence.
- Overall cost: including medical cost not covered by insurance, uncompensated time away from work, and support you will need at home. Be realistic. Consider near-term and long-term costs.

## Step 3: Respect Your Preferences

Often laying out the pros and cons in Step 2 makes the right choice plainly obvious. If a young boy fractures his wrist, "what matters most" is simple: maintain normal growth and function of his arm and hand. The theoretical options include doing nothing or splinting his arm, but the only rational option is casting it because immobilizing the joint is the only option that ensures that his bones will heal properly. A good outcome far outweighs the four to six weeks of inconvenience. In other situations, the decision is straightforward.

What if a teenage girl has scoliosis—a curvature of her spine—that puts her at risk for chronic back pain, disability, and breathing difficulties? With moderately severe scoliosis, there is often a choice between surgery and a back brace. Surgery involves a six- to ten-inch incision and implanting hardware—screws or rods—into the spine to stabilize the vertebrae; full recovery can take up to a year. The alternative option is a back brace that must be worn eighteen to twenty hours a day until she is done growing. While both approaches avoid the consequences of a twisted S- or C-shaped spine, there is not one best treatment. The best choice for a teenager rests on whether she is willing to wear the brace during the majority of the day for several years.

Identifying "what matters most" during a healthcare decision means clarifying your priorities and preferences. The simple difference is that priorities are what you consider most important whereas preferences are what you like most. Sometimes they overlap but other times they conflict and making a decision means finding a compromise. In the example below, Grace's priority was to get screened for colon cancer, but her preferences were holding her back.

Facebook Question

*Grace: It's time for me to get my colon checked. Age fifty seems to be a fun year. I have a problem with needles and having a tube so far in me concerns me.*

*Dr. Georgiou: The gold standard test for colon cancer screening is a colonoscopy. Yes, it requires an IV (needle) and there is a long tube. But, doctors use medication to keep you relaxed during the procedure. If you are still scared, you can talk to your doctor about using a medication called propofol that will put you completely "out" for a short period of time, and you won't remember a thing. If you remain so frightened that you are tempted to avoid the test completely, then there are other options for screening for colon cancer. They are not as sensitive for finding polyps or cancer, but something is better than nothing.*

Thirty-five percent of Americans ages fifty to seventy-five have not been screened for colon cancer even though the majority have health insurance that will cover the procedure.[10] For 20 percent of these unscreened people, the primary barrier is fear,[11] but Grace's willingness to express her fear of needles and long tubes helped identify screening alternatives that she would be willing to act on.

Priorities and preferences are powerful drivers of health behavior, but articulating them can make you feel vulnerable. You may judge yourself or fear being judged by others for having preferences that seem superficial, silly, shortsighted, or selfish. However, being honest with yourself, your family, and especially your doctor about what's important to you is critical in designing the healthcare solutions that are best for you. Start by having a private heart-to-heart conversation with yourself.

For Step 3, clarify "what matters most." Start by establishing your priorities:

- How do you want your life improved by this treatment/decision?
- Why are you considering a healthcare intervention? Think beyond the answer "to get better" or "to be healthy."

Then identify your preferences:

- On a scale of 0–10, how much medical risk are you willing to take to achieve your goal? (0 means you are unwilling to take any risk; 10 means that you are willing accept death as a risk.)
- On a scale of 0–10, how willing are you to tolerate a short-term restriction in your quality of life (inconvenience, pain, social/emotional impact, disability) to achieve your goal? (0 means you are unwilling to tolerate any quality-of-life restriction; 10 means that you are willing accept significant quality-of-life restriction.)
- On a scale of 0–10, how willing are you to tolerate a long-term limitation on your quality of life (permanent disability, physical deformity, ongoing social/emotional impact) to achieve your goal? (0 means you are unwilling to tolerate any long-term quality-of-life limitation; 10 means that you are willing accept significant quality-of-life limitation.)
- On a scale of 0–10, how much of a financial commitment are you willing to make to achieve your goal? (0 means you are unwilling or unable to pay anything to achieve your goal; 10 means that you are willing and able to accept full financial responsibility.)
- On a scale of 0–10, how much of a role, if any, do your cultural or religious beliefs have in your healthcare decision? Are there treatments that are prohibited by your beliefs?

These questions elicit how much you are willing to sacrifice to achieve your goals. Your answers are neither right nor wrong. They are personal. When couples are told that their unborn baby may have Down Syndrome, their decision to have advanced blood tests versus amniocentesis is highly influenced by their willingness to accept a small risk of miscarriage associated with introducing a needle into the amniotic sac. For men with early stage prostate cancer, deciding between prostatectomy, radiation, or radioactive seed implants usually revolves around the risk of incontinence, impotence, and the impact on their quality of life. Some women with breast cancer have borderline evidence of metastases and doctors give them the option of having chemotherapy after surgery; a few forego treatment based on the cost.

Most of us prefer to protect our health and well-being, quality of life, and financial stability. In idealistic decision-making situations, we can have it all without any risk or threat to our core values. Real life, however, forces trade-offs. Combining the alternatives from Step 2 with "what matters most" from Step 3 sets the stage for evaluating your options and making a fully informed decision.

## Step 4: Evaluate Your Options

Evaluating your options and landing on a decision is not a linear process. Rather, these considerations are iterative, sometimes seeming circular or repetitive as you revisit your options before making a final choice. Healthcare decisions that are the most serious aren't necessarily those that are the most difficult to make. Imagine a young mother diagnosed with a rapidly debilitating neurologic disease. If her death is imminent, it is not difficult to accept the risk of a life-threatening, painful experimental procedure if there is even a remote chance for a cure. Similarly, someone with a severe flare of ulcerative colitis, unresponsive to medications, may not have to think too long before agreeing to a colostomy in order to avoid the risk of a ruptured intestine and fatal infection. Life-threatening circumstances tend to have clear, compelling consequences. It's the choices in between that require more deliberation.

Facebook Question

*Melissa: I am thirty-seven with tonsillar stones. Is there any way to get rid of them without tonsil removal? My breath is deadly and my husband won't kiss me. I pop them out as much as I can, and try scraping my tongue and gargling, but nothing keeps them from coming back.*

*Dr. Georgiou: Melissa, this problem is causing a significant quality-of-life issue. Have you seen an ear, nose, and throat doctor? The methods you've tried are the first line of attack, but if they have failed, you may want to consider having a tonsillectomy.*

*Melissa: Surgery is the last resort thing I want to do since my age puts me at a higher risk.*

Tonsillar stones can cause halitosis (very bad breath), but don't pose a significant medical risk. However, the treatment, tonsillectomy, has a one in twenty risk of postoperative hemorrhage. Melissa was walking an emotional tightrope as she was trying to identify a solution that would allow her to maintain a healthy relationship with her husband without risking her health. Unlike Steps 1 through 3, Step 4 is more art than science. These decisions are not easy. Balancing the pros and cons in Step 2 with your priorities and preferences in Step 3 can guide you toward the right decision. While you don't want to make misguided decisions based on intuition, a well-informed decision that respects your preferences must also intuitively "feel" right so that you can sleep at night.

For Step 4, build a bridge to your decision:

- Focus on each option in Step 2 and ask: "Do the short- and long-term advantages address my priorities?" Remember to consider the option of doing nothing and set aside options that don't meet your goals.
- For each remaining option, ask: "Am I willing to accept the short- and long-term medical risks?" Set aside options where the risk is a showstopper.
- For each remaining option, ask: "Am I capable of living with the short- and long-term quality-of-life trade-offs?" Set aside options with trade-offs that are unrealistic for you to accommodate.
- For each remaining option, ask: "Am I willing and able to accept the financial responsibility?"
- For each remaining option, ask: "Will I be able to sleep at night without regret, knowing I made the right choice for me?"

If the decision is not clear after you go through the questions, take the time to refine your priorities and your preferences. Dig deeper into "what matters most" by being more specific about the outcomes you hope for and the impact you can prepare yourself for. In healthcare situations that warrant shared decision making between you and your physician, don't delay your research "to see what the doctor says." My recommendation is to work through the CARES model on your own *before* you have an in-depth discussion with your doctor. This gives you the time and the freedom to immerse yourself in the facts (about your condition) and your feelings (about your priorities and preferences) so that you can fully participate in the conversation with your doctor when you meet to discuss your options.

Remember, in any meeting, the person with the agenda controls the meeting, and every meeting needs an agenda. Whether it's a strategy session at work or a planning meeting for a dinner party with friends, having an agenda keeps the meeting focused and ensures that key issues are addressed. An office visit with your doctor to discuss a healthcare decision is a meeting—and let me be clear—it's *your* meeting about *your* health. So invest time preparing for the meeting and then lead it. This will help assure that both you and your doctor have a chance to discuss issues that are important.

Type a brief but formal agenda with bullet points for each of the discussion topics you want to cover. The agenda template below follows the CARES model and is a logical sequence for any shared decision-making visit.

Agenda

- Understanding of my condition.
- Treatment alternatives, pros and cons.
- My priorities and preferences.
- Discussion.
- Other questions and concerns.

Make two copies of the agenda; give one to the doctor and start the conversation by saying, "There is a lot of information to cover today. It would help me to go through the items on this list so that all my questions are answered and so that you give me your best advice." Use your notes and worksheets from Steps 1 through 4 of the CARES model to discuss each bullet point (for example, "Here is my understanding of my condition and why I need treatment." "Here is a list of the treatment alternatives along with the pros and cons.").

Giving a doctor insight to your knowledge, assumptions, and point of view is just as diagnostic and therapeutic as the results from your most recent lab test or x-ray. While unconventional (and a bit scary for some readers), most doctors welcome this approach. Interacting with an engaged patient and gauging what they know and how they feel allows the doctor to personalize the treatment plan to you and your needs.

Think about how much more effective it is having your doctor:

- Skip over the basics (if you already know them) and dedicate meeting time to deepening your understanding of the condition. Ask your doctor to address misunderstandings you may have.
- Clarify the pros and cons of the treatment alternatives and have a conversation about how the details of your medical situation affect the likelihood of advantages, disadvantages, and risk of complications.
- Understand what's important so your doctor can deliberate with you, based on your priorities and preferences.
- Avoid thought traps that could lead to bad decisions by addressing any misguided perceptions and biases you have shared with your doctor.
- Hear and address issues and concerns that are causing you distress.

What if you don't have time to become well informed? What if you find yourself in a doctor's office or the emergency room when you hear, for the very first time, that you need an invasive procedure, surgery, or medication? With the exception of an emergency intervention to save your life, a limb, or your functional capacity, you should never feel rushed to make a decision to accommodate the time limitations of a medical office visit, the physician's workload, or the operating room schedule. Even in an urgent situation, it is reasonable to demand a few hours to think through and review all your options. In a nonurgent situation, state that you need some time to review all your options; and to avoid having your care fall through the cracks, schedule a follow-up appointment before you leave the office that day. Giving yourself time to independently evaluate your options protects you from a type of brain paralysis that can occur when your doctor offers his or her "expert" opinion. Neurobiologic research and brain scans show that when people are given expert advice, the decision-making parts of the brain often shut down. The risk is that you ignore your own internal value mechanisms and offload the decision making to the expert. [12]

## Step 5: Start Taking Action

A common coping mechanism after making a major healthcare decision is to "take one day at a time." This mindset can relieve some short-term anxiety, but reinforces a passive relationship with the physician and fuels a lack of accountability to your care plan. Alternatively, understanding "what's next?" and what you have to do empowers you to communicate with the physician, ask the *right* questions, and be assertive about your needs.

For Step 5, create a calendar and a detailed roadmap for your care:

- What (exactly) do you have to do over the next thirty, sixty, and ninety days?
- What side effects can you expect?
- What are the indicators that show that this treatment plan is working or not working?

Make sure that you understand how your life—work, activities, energy, sex, driving—will be different. Plan for it. If there is an aspect of the regimen that isn't compatible with your life and lifestyle, speak up and negotiate a more compatible approach. Understand when bumps in the road can be safely addressed at home and when they are serious enough to require medical attention. Anticipating complications may feel scary, but preparation arms you with information that can prevent overreacting, getting discouraged, or feeling tethered to a 24/7 lifeline with the physician. Finally, have the courage to discuss "what's next?" if your healthcare course is not progressing as expected. Know when it is time to reconsider your options.

## NOTES

1. M. Viswanathan et al., "Interventions to Improve Adherence to Self-Administered Medications for Chronic Diseases in the United States: A Systematic Review," *Annals of Internal Medicine* 157 (2012): 785–95.

2. J. L. Cataldo et al., "The Use of Compression Stockings for Venous Disorders in Brazil," *Phlebology: The Journal of Venous Disease* 27, no. 1 (2012): 33–37, doi:10.1258/phleb.2011.010088.

3. A. Brown, "Evaluating the Reasons Underlying Treatment Nonadherence in VLU Patients: Mishel's Theory of Uncertainty: Part 2 of 2," *Journal of Wound Care* 23, no. 2 (February 2014): 73–80.

4. John Weinman et al., "How Accurate Is Patients' Anatomical Knowledge: A Cross-Sectional, Questionnaire Study of Six Patient Groups and a

General Public Sample," *BMC Family Practice* 10, no. 43 (2009): doi:10.1186/1471-2296-10-43.

5. "Gunther von Hagens' Body Worlds: The Original Exhibition of Real Human Bodies," accessed October 21, 2015, http://www.bodyworlds.com/en/exhibitions/past_exhibitions.html.

6. Peter Leiberich et al., "Body Worlds Exhibition—Visitor Attitudes and Emotions," *Annals of Anatomy* 188, no. 6 (November 14, 2006): 567–73.

7. Paul Scullard et al., "Googling Children's Health: Reliability of Medical Advice on the Internet," *Archives of Disease in Childhood* 95 (April 6, 2010): 580–82, doi:10.1136/adc.2009.168856.

8. B. J. Fogg et al., "How Do Users Evaluate the Credibility of Web Sites? A Study with Over 2,500 Participants," accessed October 23, 2015, http://htlab.psy.unipd.it/uploads/Pdf/lectures/captology/p1-fogg.pdf.

9. Jakob Nielsen, "How Long Do Users Stay on Web Pages?" *NN/g Nielsen Norman Group*, September 12, 2011, accessed October 27, 2015, http://www.nngroup.com/articles/how-long-do-users-stay-on-web-pages.

10. "Colorectal Cancer Screening Rates Remain Low," *Centers for Disease Control and Prevention*, November 5, 2013, http://www.cdc.gov/media/releases/2013/p1105-colorectal-cancer-screening.html.

11. R. M. Jones et al., "Patient-Reported Barriers to Colorectal Cancer Screening: A Mixed-Methods Analysis," *American Journal of Preventive Medicine* 38, no. 5 (2010): 508–16, doi:10.1016/j.amepre.2010.01.021.

12. Jan B. Engelmann et al., "Expert Financial Advice Neurobiologically 'Offloads' Financial Decision-Making Under Risk," *Public Library of Science ONE* 4, no. 3 (March 24, 2009): doi:10.1371/journal.pone.0004957.

# 5

# SORTING THROUGH ALTERNATIVE CARE

**F**acebook Question

*Margie: I have a granddaughter who is three years old. She has ITP. Are there any natural herbs that would help with this issue? I would like some options.*

*Dr. Georgiou: Margie, you didn't mention whether the ITP is a new or ongoing condition for your granddaughter, so I will assume that it is acute (new), which is the most common. Here's the good news about acute ITP: it usually resolves in a few weeks though it could take up to six months. And, in the meantime (this is the bad news), she is at risk for bleeding—from her gums, from small cuts, from her urine or stool, or into her brain—since she doesn't have enough platelets to form clots. While you asked me about herbs that may help, the most important information I can give you is to make sure your granddaughter is being closely followed by a hematologist. What you can do for her is to make sure that she stays safe and avoids getting injured when she is playing. This is a serious condition and not one where you want to experiment with herbs or other unproven treatments.*

ITP refers to idiopathic (unknown cause) thrombocytopenic (low platelets) purpura (bruises caused by bleeding from small blood vessels). Acute ITP in children frequently follows a cold or viral infection, presumably because the body creates antibodies to fight the virus and then gets confused and mistakenly creates antibodies that destroy the body's platelets. Some children don't need treatment for ITP, but when treatment is necessary (which happens when their platelets are dangerously low), the most common treatments are steroids (like prednisone) or intravenous infusions of antibodies. There are no proven herbal therapies for ITP.

I didn't know whether Margie's granddaughter was being seen by a specialist or whether she was even stable. Without knowing the details, my concern was that Margie's focus on herbal remedies for such a serious condition might be distracting her from getting the child the care she needed. Because a delay could be life threatening, I didn't mince any words and took a strong position, steering her back to the physician and away from unconventional, and in this case unproven, treatment.

Margie's question was not wrong or inappropriate. As I emphasized in chapter 4, knowing all the possible treatment options is an important step in making decisions. The key is identifying proven complementary and alternative medicine therapies while dismissing remedies that are unproven and lack any health benefit. This chapter will teach you how to use the CARES model to consider effective, though still unconventional, options in your decision-making process.

About 5 percent of the questions I get on Facebook are from viewers who want my opinion, guidance, or reassurance about a "natural," "holistic," "alternative," or "herbal" treatment for their condition. There are many terms used to describe alternative practices. Complementary and Alternative Medicine (CAM) and Integrative Medicine are two commonly used catch-all terms for healthcare approaches developed outside of mainstream science-based medicine. These terms encompass a wide range of practices and products such as herbal supplements, meditation, traditional Chinese medicine, energy practices, chiropractic, acupuncture, and naturopathy. Americans embrace alternative practices; more than 30 percent of adults and almost 12 percent of children use alternative approaches[1] to enhance their general health and well-being and to treat musculoskeletal conditions.

Sometimes there is solid scientific evidence that a particular therapy works. Chiropractic has been shown to be effective in treating acute low back pain. Melatonin can ease sleeplessness. Mindfulness training has helped people to cope with irritable bowel syndrome. On the other hand, consumers spend the most money on the "nonvitamin, nonmineral, dietary supplement" category of CAM therapies such as fish oil (for "heart health"), glucosamine (for "healthy joints"), and echinacea and ginseng (to "boost" the immune system)[2]—even though the benefits are unclear. Sixty-five percent of people with cancer have pursued some complementary approaches to help them manage cancer symptoms or treatment side effects and improve their quality of life,[3] even though no alternative health product or practice has ever been proven to cure cancer. Practitioner-based alternative services such as chiropractic, massage, acupuncture, and energy healing are generally not supported or recommended by physicians. Despite all this, Americans spend $33.9 *billion* out of pocket each year for these therapies.[4]

So what motivates patients to pursue and use unconventional services in the absence of good evidence of efficacy or recommendation by their doctor? Studies show that the people most likely to use CAM have conditions with substantial pain, lack of a definitive cure, and an unpredictable prognosis.[5] Back pain affects 80 percent of the population at some time during their lifetime and is the most common condition treated using nonmainstream therapies.[6] People with cancer, however, are the most likely group to look beyond traditional science-based medicine for their care. Studies show that patients who select alternative therapies feel a greater sense of control.[7] They tend to believe in the "holistic"—mind, body, spirit—philosophy offered by CAM practitioners. They believe in the body's innate ability to heal itself and are less comfortable depending solely on medical science-based treatments. They also want to be active participants in their care. They feel comfortable self-prescribing supplements that can be purchased without a prescription and making appointments with alternative practitioners without needing to get "permission," or referrals, from their medical physicians. CAM users want to feel empowered.

However, a traditional medical treatment must be evaluated based on whether it is the right treatment for the right person at the right time for the right condition, and nonmainstream treatments should be held to the same standards. Frequently, though, perceptions about alternative treatments can kidnap and mask facts, causing people to accept these treatments without evaluating them as carefully. Here are some of the most common thought traps:

- *"It's natural, so it's safe."* Properly used, many herbal products are safe but "natural" does not guarantee that everything on the supplement shelf is innocuous. There are "natural" products that may interact with prescribed medications or increase the risk of liver or kidney toxicity or bleeding. Loose regulatory standards means that products can often contain contaminants or don't contain the ingredient printed on the label at all. In 2015, four national retailers selling popular supplements such as echinacea, ginseng, and St. John's Wort were sent cease and desist letters by New York's attorneys general. Overall, 79 percent of the chains' store brand herbal supplement labels did not reflect the actual ingredients. For example, in one store, in pills labeled ginkgo biloba, the substance in the bottle was rice, asparagus, and spruce.[8] This deception poses a particularly high risk to people with food allergies. The distorted perception that natural products are risk free is fueled by health food store personnel who have limited training and do not consistently highlight side effects with customers.[9]
- *"My friend swears by it."* An influential source of information for CAM treatments is the personal experience of enthusiastic family, friends, and acquaintances[10]—especially when people relate stories of success after conventional treatments have failed. Parents of a colicky baby, for example, are particularly vulnerable to advice because there is no definitive medical or alternative treatment for an inconsolable infant. Exasperated and desperate for relief, some parents resort to trying chiropractic manipulation and naturopathy because it "worked" for other parents with a similar experience. Among men with prostate cancer who use unconventional treatments, the personal (anecdotal) stories of patients who have been helped by CAM serve as the "evidence" of effectiveness.[11]
- *"It's been around for thousands of years."* Many cultures have healing traditions—ranging from acupuncture to prayer—without solid evidence that they work. The absence of science is not a reason to discard the experiences of previous generations. At the same time, history does not make these practices immune to scientific analysis. When objective evidence *is* available that supports or disputes the effectiveness or safety, it is important to consider these facts in the decision-making process. For example, acupunc-

ture rarely causes harm. However, when not delivered properly, acupuncture has caused serious adverse effects, including infections from nonsterile needles, punctured organs, collapsed lungs, and injury to the central nervous system.

## CONVENTIONAL VERSUS ALTERNATIVE

The goals of physicians and alternative practitioners are similar: both want to maintain and restore health. However, their approaches are as different as yin and yang. A key difference is the process by which patients are diagnosed. Medical physicians use patients' symptoms as a guide to help them identify and target the specific microscopic anatomic structures or biochemical processes causing those symptoms. Eliminating the disease is the top priority, which explains why traditional medicine uses chemotherapy to kill cancer cells, antibiotics to kill bacteria, and surgery to remove damaged tissue. Alternative practitioners, on the other hand, focus on eliminating symptoms. They embrace the belief that health is synonymous with balance, and they use symptoms as a guide to identify the body's overall imbalance. Instead of removing disease, CAM therapies are based on the belief that focusing on energy fields and the body's natural defense mechanisms can return the body to a balanced state.

Facebook Question

*Kathy: What is a natural herb one can use for menopause? Any help would be greatly appreciated.*

*Dr. Georgiou: Kathy, what aspect of menopause are you concerned about? Are you concerned about preventing osteoporosis? Getting rid of flashes? Vaginal dryness? Other symptoms?*

Kathy didn't respond, but I will assume she had hot flashes because this is the most common complaint among women going through menopause. A CAM provider is most likely to suggest yoga, tai chi, qi gong, or acupuncture. There is some research showing that these practices decrease the frequency and intensity of the hot flashes, presumably by reducing stress. Alternative providers may also suggest black cohash, an herb that might decrease hot flashes by having an estrogen-like effect on the body.

A gynecologist hearing her symptoms will most likely start by verifying that the root cause of her symptoms is, indeed, menopause-related. He will do blood tests to evaluate FSH and LH levels. High levels of these hormones in the blood are biochemical signs that the ovaries are not producing estrogen. A gynecologist will also think beyond treating the symptoms and order a bone density test, knowing that a silent but dangerous complication of estrogen deficiency is osteoporosis. Once the diagnosis is established, a common recommendation is hormone replacement therapy. This therapy resupplies the body with the estrogen and progesterone hormones it no longer produces, protects her bones, and reduces her hot flash symptoms.

Kathy could benefit from using *both* the mind-body practices (yoga, tai chi, etc.) and hormone replacement therapy. Some unconventional treatments have been shown to address the symptoms by reducing stress; the hormone treatment targets the biological basis of the symptoms. This combined approach, using nonmainstream practices *together* with conventional medicine, is a "complementary" approach to care. People often use "alternative" and "complementary" interchangeably, but these terms refer to different concepts. "Alternative" treatments are nonmainstream practices used as a *substitute* for conventional therapy; most people pursue them without their physician's knowledge. The potential danger is that an alternative treatment, used exclusively, may resolve symptoms and help a patient feel "healthy"—even though silent disease, or risk of disease, may still be lurking in the body.

## Facebook Question

*Nicole: Are white mulberry dietary supplements beneficial for your sugar levels in your body?*

*Dr. Georgiou: White mulberry is an herb commonly used by Chinese traditional medicine practitioners to help control blood sugar. There are chemicals in white mulberry that slow the break down of sugars so they are more slowly absorbed and help keep blood sugar in a normal range. While white mulberry is not a mainstream treatment in the United States, there are some small published studies showing that it might be an option for some people with diabetes. However, you shouldn't treat yourself. Discuss this option with your doctor. Finally, if you do use this herb, it is important to monitor your blood glucose just as you would if you were on a prescription oral diabetes medication or insulin.*

I confess. When I refreshed the chat site and Nicole's question popped up, I thought, "How ridiculous. An herb for diabetes?" My 1980s Johns Hopkins education was steeped in traditional science-based medicine, and the conventional way to treat high blood sugar is diet, exercise, oral hypoglycemic medications, and insulin—not herbs. Fortunately, I caught myself in my own bias and did some quick research before answering. I surprised myself when I found several studies about white mulberry, including one showing that taking the powder three times daily for four weeks decreased fasting blood glucose by about 27 percent in patients with type 2 diabetes.[12] This was a good reminder to me that science does not have geographic boundaries. I directed Nicole back to her doctor because this Chinese therapy seemed to have some valid scientific evidence behind it and was an alternative worth considering.

After I responded, I needed to satisfy my own curiosity. I did some additional online research about this herb and learned that the handful of human studies were small, the majority of the studies were conducted in rats, and the long-term safety of taking white mulberry is unclear. White mulberry might work, but it might not. In short, there just wasn't enough credible scientific research to know one way or the other. Would I recommend or "prescribe" this treatment to a patient with high blood sugar if I were a mainstream practicing physician? No. I would also not prescribe any drug before its efficacy was supported by credible scientific evidence. Limited scientific evidence is a legitimate barrier to most physicians' promoting or endorsing alternative medicine treatments.[13] And frankly, the liability risk is too high. However, I would support a patient who opens the discussion about this herbal treatment, understands the limitations of the studies, accepts the potential risks, and advocates for a closely monitored trial of white mulberry herbs instead of prescription medication.

Archelle's Insider Tip
*Educate yourself then share the information with your physician.*
*Studies show that doctors are most likely to refer patients to CAM*
*therapies when patients initiate the request.* [14]

Finding objective information about alternative therapies is even more
challenging than finding credible information about medical treatments. A Google search for information about a medical therapy re-
turns at least one or two credible sites in the top search results. The
search results for alternative therapies are more likely to bring up marketing websites promoting alternative providers and products. For example, in my search for information on "reiki," my top results included:

- Six websites for local reiki providers.
- Two "professional" sites promoting reiki providers.
- Two websites focused on medical quackery.
- One website with ratings and reviews of local reiki providers.
- One dictionary site defining reiki.
- One site affiliated with an academic medical center and medical
  school.

Websites that promise "balance," "healing," and "increasing the life
force energy" are intriguing. However, twelve of the thirteen sites on
the first page of search results were biased, promotional sites and only
the university-sponsored site offered objective information. These
twelve sites had one or more of the four "red flags" that should make
you highly suspicious of a site:

- Products available for online purchasing.
- Patient testimonials.
- Descriptions of the CAM treatment as a "cure."
- Promotion of treatments as "having no side effects." [15]

Being the arbiter of credible CAM treatment sites is especially difficult
because the entire field of unconventional treatments has fewer standards, regulations, and guidelines than conventional medicine. Because
I prefer to spend more time learning rather than vetting websites, I rely
on three "go to" sites for credible evidence about unconventional options.

- For general information: The National Center for Complementary and Integrative Health (NCCIH) is a division of the National Institutes of Health (NIH) and focuses on funding scientific research on alternative medicine and making that information available to clinicians and to the public.[16] The "A to Z" health information on the NCCIH (nccih.nih.gov) site gives a balanced overview of a wide range of herbs used as alternative therapies. It also identifies nonmainstream treatments that complement traditional approaches for a broad range of conditions from allergies and acne to wound care and warts.
- For cancer-related CAM treatment information: With 47 percent of cancer patients using alternative therapies in addition to conventional treatment,[17] NIH has a separate site, The Office of Cancer Complementary and Alternative Medicine (cam.cancer.gov), that focuses exclusively on treatments related to the diagnosis, prevention, and treatment of cancer.
- For detailed information on unconventional treatments: The Cochrane Complementary Medicine website (cam.cochrane.org), based at the University of Maryland Center for Integrative Medicine, includes almost 250 Cochrane Reviews about alternative therapies. These reviews are considered an unbiased "gold standard" by physicians because the authors inventory and summarize the research findings from *all* the well-conducted published studies on a specific alternative therapy topic.

## USING CARES FOR COMPLEMENTARY AND ALTERNATIVE TREATMENTS

Chapter 4 explained how to use the CARES model to make the right care choices for your health and healthcare. However, considering CAM treatments in addition to, or instead of, traditional therapies should not be a separate or parallel process. You should consider all of your alternatives as part of a single, holistic decision about your care. Because your doctor might not be knowledgeable about these treatments, there are some additional steps you need to take in the CARES process to help assure that you and your doctor are well informed and making the right decision.

## Step 1: Understand Your Condition

Science-based medicine uses medications and surgeries to target a specific biologic process. For example, if you have hypertension-related headaches, successful treatment starts with decreasing your blood pressure to put less strain on your heart muscle. Understanding the anatomy and physiology of your condition is the foundation for decision making, and the long-term risk of developing heart disease is the "so what?" Alternative medicine, however, focuses on improving your health experience; alleviating the headache (rather than lowering the blood pressure) is the priority. Understanding what you might *feel* during the course of your condition is the starting point for considering nonmainstream treatments.

You accomplished the basics for this step in chapter 4. The overview of your condition in your "go to" credible health information website outlined the most common symptoms of the condition and complications of the treatments and procedures. However, symptoms—especially stress, pain, and fatigue—are personal. What you feel and experience is influenced by your physical condition—but your emotional, social, and financial well-being also play powerful roles. Therefore a website summary cannot completely predict the extent to which symptoms might be bothersome to you. For example, I know many women who had radiation therapy for breast cancer. Some didn't notice side effects at all and simply incorporated the radiation treatment into their workday. Others were so fatigued that they stopped working for the five to six weeks that they were receiving treatments. Why the difference? The most common psychological cause of cancer-related fatigue is emotional stress.[18] Fifteen to 25 percent of patients who have cancer also experience depression, but in this instance, the clinical definition of depression may not tell the whole story. Emotional symptoms can have an impact on quality of life even if they are subtle and don't meet the criteria for a psychiatric diagnosis. Illness can change your outlook toward your family, your work, and your kids. It can affect your motivation. It can eat away at your self-confidence and your sense of hope for the future.

Understanding how a condition may affect your emotional well-being and quality of life sets the stage for identifying alternative treatments that can help. Joining a support group, whether online or in person, can connect you with people facing similar issues. Studies show that one of the primary benefits of these groups is that participants are better informed about their illness and have a clearer understanding of what to expect because members of support groups often share experiences. In addition to being a resource for information, support groups can function as a complement to medical treatment. Across a broad range of conditions, these groups support a medical treatment plan by helping patients cope and manage the effects of the condition on you and your relationships.[19]

Your doctor, the Internet, advocacy organizations, or people with the same condition can be sources to help you identify support groups. However, be sure to be read the "community rules" of a group before joining or posting any information. Be selective. Make sure that the group has clear processes that maintain your confidentiality. A good rule of thumb is to look for groups with a layperson or health professional acting as a moderator. This will keep the conversation threads focused on relevant topics and help assure that the conversation content is not misleading or harmful. At first, it may seem like a fire hose of scary information, but the support group community will give you real-life insight into the full range of symptoms that may occur.

For Step 1, focus on the symptoms that are most likely to be part of *your* experience.

- List the symptoms you currently have that are associated with your condition.
- List the symptoms (side effects) that you are most likely to experience as a result of the treatment. For example, if you have major surgery, you will predictably have pain. Certain types of chemotherapy almost always cause hair loss; others cause nausea.
- What symptom(s) are you most afraid of? Why does it scare you? How will this symptom(s) disrupt your quality of life?

## Step 2: Know Your Alternatives

Susan Carstens taught me the importance of preserving quality of life. In November 2011, Susan saw her doctor for what she thought was just some back pain. Instead, she was diagnosed with metastatic ovarian cancer and quickly entered the world of traditional medicine with a care team that included oncologists, gynecologic surgeons, pathologists, and radiologists. Although she had a radical hysterectomy, radiation therapy, and chemotherapy, Susan was not naïve about her prognosis. The five-year survival rate for advanced ovarian cancer, despite treatment, is abysmal—between 17 and 39 percent.[20] What concerned Susan even more than dying were the potential side effects of her chemotherapy. Cisplatin is one of the most common agents used to treat solid tumors. It is effective because it interferes with the DNA of cancer cells and keeps them from multiplying. Unfortunately, cisplatin also interferes with the DNA of healthy cells. Severe nausea and vomiting are predictable side effects, but Susan was more concerned with the neurotoxic side effects of the chemotherapy. By day, Susan worked as a juvenile specialist with the local police department in Minnesota. In her spare time, she was a ballroom dancer and she was most afraid that numbness, tingling, and pain in her feet might keep her from doing what she loved most. Susan was fortunate to have a surgeon who referred her to the complementary and alternative services team at the hospital. Several small studies have shown that acupuncture improves nerve symptoms in cancer-related neuropathy.[21] Within a few weeks of her surgery, Susan's treatment plan included regular acupuncture sessions.

I met Susan when I interviewed her for a KSTP health special in February 2015. The weekly acupuncture sessions over four years helped decrease the symptoms in her feet; she was still taking dance lessons and competing. As Susan shared her medical story, I sensed that the end was near and my eyes welled up with tears. But Susan just smiled and told me that dancing the fox trot, waltz, tango, and bolero throughout her illness helped her keep a positive attitude so that she could live one day at a time.

For Step 2, search the "go to" sites for alternative treatments for the symptoms and/or side effects you are most concerned about. Answer the following questions:

- Are there alternative treatments that can be used to treat your symptoms?
- What evidence exists that each of these treatments works to alleviate the symptom(s)?

Then expand the chart from the "Know Your Alternatives" section of chapter 4 to summarize the advantages and disadvantages of the non-traditional alternatives you are considering. Pay special attention to whether the alternative treatments interfere with or compromise the conventional medical care you are/will be receiving. Be sure to compare alternative treatments with the conventional medicine alternatives that are available to treat your symptoms. Finally, call your insurance company to determine the cost of alternative treatments. Don't guess or make assumptions. What they cover is complex and confusing because insurance rules vary depending on state laws, regulations, and differences among specific insurance plans. Questions to ask include:[22]

- Is this complementary approach covered for my health condition?
- Does it need to be preauthorized or preapproved?
- Do I need a referral from my doctor?
- Are there any limits on the number of visits or the amount you will pay?

## Steps 3 and 4: Respect Your Preferences; Evaluate Your Options

"What matters most" when considering CAM means identifying the therapies that can help you *feel* healthy—even when you aren't. In Step 1, you already identified your highest priority, the symptom you would most like to eliminate or minimize to maintain your quality of life.

The focus in Step 3 is to identify your preferences and the trade-offs you are willing to make to receive the benefit of a nonmainstream service. Like all decisions, the process is a balancing act.

Your preferences are likely very different for alternative treatments than for medical treatments. You may be willing to tolerate uncomfortable symptoms and even the risk of long-term complications from medical therapies in order to eradicate biologic disease. However, because the goal of CAM treatments is to improve your experience during treatment, unconventional options should not impose *more* pain, discomfort, complications, adverse reactions, or long-term risk. Yes, this is a personal decision that you must make for yourself; however, my recommendation is to eliminate any options from Step 2 that may further complicate a healthcare situation. In addition, be aware that some alternative treatment providers can foster the perception that they are treating the biological basis of your disease—even when they're not.

For the remaining treatment options on the list from Step 2, the trade-offs to consider boil down to your willingness to tolerate complexity, cost, and (in)convenience.

- Complexity: Incorporating an alternative therapy into your treatment plan increases the complexity of your care plan. It may require identifying and vetting a new practitioner and facilitating communication with your existing team. (More on that in Step 4.) Even just adding an herbal supplement to your medications may make it harder to be adherent with all your prescriptions.
- Cost: Most prescription insurance plans do not cover herbs and supplements; therefore virtually 100 percent of these costs are an out-of-pocket expense. Some practitioner-based therapies may be covered by insurance, but there is frequently a copayment or coinsurance that must be paid. On average, individuals spend about $120 per person for alternative therapies.[23]
- (In)convenience: Scheduling practitioner-based treatments means adding more appointments to your calendar and further disrupting your daily routine.

For Step 3, it's important to balance the importance of the benefits relative to the trade-offs you'll experience with a CAM therapy. Using a scale of 1–10, indicate:

- The importance of eliminating this symptom to maintain your quality of life. 1 means that it is relatively unimportant; 10 means it is so important that life may not be worth living if this symptom is present. (Benefits)
- The level of burden imposed by the complexities, cost, and (in)convenience of the CAM therapy. 1 means these three elements are not a burden; 10 means the burden exceeds what you are willing to tolerate. (Trade-offs)

How do the weights of the benefits and trade-offs compare? This simple process quantifies and clarifies your priorities and preferences. Honor them. Don't pursue any treatment with an attitude of "I might as well." Pursue treatment because it is important to your well-being.

If you decide to use an alternative treatment, don't compartmental-ize your care. Too often, patients include nonmainstream therapies into their care plan without sharing this information with their physician. One study showed that even among people who were actively seeing a physician, between 63 percent and 72 percent of patients did not dis-close their use of alternative therapies during their visits because:[24]

- *"It wasn't important for the doctor to know."* (61 percent)
- *"The doctor never asked."* (60 percent)
- *"It's none of the doctor's business."* (31 percent)
- *"The doctor would not understand."* (20 percent)

However, the majority of physicians (74 percent) is supportive, concep-tually, of complementary therapies and believes that clinical care *should* integrate the best conventional and alternative practices so that patients benefit from the full range of proven physical, emotional, mental, so-cial, and spiritual approaches that affect a patient's health condition.[25] It is also true that a much lower percentage, fewer than 50 percent, actually recommends and refers patients to CAM therapies.[26] One rea-son for this gap is that doctors are self-aware (but may not readily admit) that their reluctance to support nonmainstream treatments stems from their own lack of knowledge. They are interested in helping their patients make informed decisions about alternative treatments, but most do not feel qualified to have the discussion.[27] Other physicians may be concerned about unorthodox therapies that are not supported by scientific evidence. Don't slip into being passive aggressive. If this is important to you, you need to take the first step. Involve your physician and ask for his or her input as you evaluate your options to help assure that your care is safe and coordinated. You expect a physician to support conventional treatments based on credible scientific evidence; likewise, you should expect them to only support evidence-based alternative therapies.

## Archelle's Insider Tip
*The language and approach you use to discuss an alternative treat-ment with your doctor will determine whether they respond defensively or collaboratively. Getting your doctor to listen and care during a con-*

*versation about unconventional options means having a strategy to overcome time constraints and insecurity.*

- *Start by appealing to their emotional side. "I am really afraid." Focus on the specific symptoms and how they will affect your quality of life.*
- *Then engage their intellect. "What recommendations do you have for dealing with these symptoms?" Who knows? They may offer additional alternatives that you are not aware of.*
- *Finally, educate with data. "There is evidence that meditation (deep breathing, ginger, reiki therapy, etc.) helps these symptoms." Share the information you have gathered from credible websites along with your summary of the advantages, disadvantages, and your preferences.*

### Step 5: Start Taking Action

Your physician's support does not ensure that he or she can or will actively help you coordinate alternative therapies into your care plan. First, your physician may not know any providers to refer you to for a particular service. Because most physicians cluster together socially and professionally, they typically do not have regular referral relationships with CAM practitioners. In one study, about 65 percent of physicians recommended that their patients consult a chiropractor but only 24 percent actually made a formal referral.[28] Second, physicians say they want more communication with alternative providers who are part of the team, but get little objective feedback from their patients or the alternative provider regarding the results of nonmainstream treatments.[29]

It is important to be just as careful and thorough in your search for an alternative practitioner as you are in your search for a physician. Unfortunately, it's harder. Credentials required for complementary health practitioners vary tremendously from state to state and from discipline to discipline. For example, in some states, nutritionists[30] and naturopaths[31] do not need a license to practice.

For Step 5, identify a competent CAM practitioner.

- Call your local hospital or medical school. Ask for names of practitioners who are on the hospital staff or on the academic faculty. These alternative providers have been vetted.
- Understand your state and local government's requirements for licensing and certification of practitioners and the limitations of those requirements. The easiest way to find this information is by searching "(State) licensure requirements for (Alternative Provider)" (for example, "Minnesota licensure requirements for naturopaths").
- Verify the licensure status of any provider before your first visit. Many states have an online "license look-up" function on their regulatory board's website. Use it.
- Update all of your physicians and practitioners about the progress of your care plan.

It takes some effort to maintain a single integrated care plan when you add a new practitioner to the mix. Enter the details about your CAM therapy visits and medications into the calendar and roadmap from chapter 4. Make sure you understand the potential side effects to watch for and document any symptoms that you experience. Most important, list the criteria you will use to decide whether the therapy is helping. After each session with your alternative provider, have the discipline to ask yourself, "Are my symptoms better as a result of this treatment?" Be objective. Take a look at the weights you applied to the risks and benefits in Step 3. Do the benefits continue to exceed the complexity, cost, and inconvenience trade-offs? If so, stay on course. If not, reevaluate your choices. Share this calendar with all your providers at each visit to give each of them full visibility to your care.

Here's the bottom line: In order to fully, and safely, benefit from both the medical and complementary aspects of your care, your level of involvement in your own care needs to be dialed to "high." You may need to do your own legwork to find a qualified practitioner and then take responsibility for keeping both sides of your treatment team fully informed.

## NOTES

1. Tainya C. Clarke, PhD, MPH, et al., "Trends in the Use of Complementary Health Approaches Among Adults: United States, 2002–2012," *National Health Statistics Reports*, no. 7 (February 10, 2015); Patricia M. Barnes, MA, et al., "Complementary and Alternative Medicine Use Among Adults and Children: United States, 2007," *National Health Statistics Reports*, no. 18 (July 30, 2009).

2. Barnes et al., "Complementary and Alternative Medicine Use Among Adults and Children."

3. National Center for Complementary and Integrative Health, accessed November 17, 2015, https://nccih.nih.gov/health/cancer/camcancer.htm.

4. "Americans Spent $33.9 Billion Out-of-Pocket on Complementary and Alternative Medicine," National Center for Complementary and Integrative Health, last modified February 20, 2013, https://nccih.nih.gov/news/2009/073009.htm.

5. "Prevalence, Cost, and Patterns of CAM Use," in *Complementary and Alternative Medicine in the United States*, Committee on the Use of Complementary and Alternative Medicine by the American Public, Board of Health Promotion and Disease Prevention (Washington, DC: National Academies Press, 2005).

6. J. K. Freburger et al., "The Rising Prevalence of Chronic Low Back Pain," *Archives of Internal Medicine* 169, no. 3 (2009): 251–58, doi:10.1001/archinternmed.2008.543.

7. Marja J. Verhoef et al., "Reasons for and Characteristics Associated with Complementary and Alternative Medicine Use Among Adult Cancer Patients: A Systematic Review," *Integrative Cancer Therapies* 4, no. 4 (December 2005): 274.

8. Eric T. Schneiderman, "Asks Major Retailers to Halt Sales of Certain Herbal Supplements As DNA Tests Fail to Detect Plant Materials Listed on Majority of Products Tested," letter to retailers, February 3, 2015, accessed April 27, 2016, http://www.ag.ny.gov/press-release/ag-schneiderman-asks-major-retailers-halt-sales-certain-herbal-supplements-dna-tests.

9. Lucy K. Helyer et al., "The Use of Complementary and Alternative Medicines Among Patients With Locally Advanced Breast Cancer—A Descriptive Study," *BMC Cancer* 6, no. 39 (February 2006), doi:10.1186/1471-2407-6-39.

10. M. Evans et al., "Decisions to Use Complementary and Alternative Medicine (CAM) by Male Cancer Patients: Information-Seeking Roles and Types of Evidence Used," *BMC Complementary Alternative Medicine* 7, no. 25 (August 4, 2007), doi:10.1186/1472-6882-7-25.

11. Ibid.

12. B. Andallu et al., "Effect of Mulberry (*Morus indica* L.) Therapy on Plasma and Erythrocyte Membrane Lipids in Patients with Type 2 Diabetes," *Clinica Chimica Acta International Journal of Clinical Chemistry and Diagnostic Laboratory Medicine* 314 (2001): 47–53.

13. "Most Doctors Not Knowledgeable About Herbals," *HealthDay News*, April 26, 2010, accessed June 15, 2010, www.modernmedicine.com/modernmedicine/Modern+Medicine+Now/Most-Doctors-Not-Knowledgeable-About-Herbals/ArticleNewsFeed/Article/detail/666928.

14. Brian M. Berman et al., "Compliance with Requests for Complementary-Alternative Medicine Referrals: A Survey of Primary Care Physicians," *Integrative Medicine* 2, no. 1 (December 1999): 11–17.

15. S. C. Matthews et al., "The Internet for Medical Information About Cancer: Help or Hindrance?" *Psychosomatics* 44 (2003): 100–103.

16. "National Institutes of Health," U.S. Department of Health and Human Services, accessed December 1, 2015, http://www.hhs.gov/about/budget/fy2015/budget-in-brief/nih/index.html.

17. N. King et al., "Surveys of Cancer Patients and Cancer Health Care Providers Regarding Complementary Therapy Use, Communication, and Information Needs," *Integrative Cancer Therapies* 14, no. 6 (November 2015): 515–24.

18. "Fatigue-Patient Version (PDQ®) Causes of Fatigue in Cancer Patients," accessed December 19, 2015, http://www.cancer.gov/about-cancer/treatment/side-effects/fatigue/fatigue-pdq#section/_27.

19. C. F. van Uden-Kraan et al., "Participation in Online Patient Support Groups Endorses Patients' Empowerment," *Patient Education and Counseling* 74, no. 1 (January 2009): 61–69.

20. "Survival Rates for Ovarian Cancer by Stage," accessed December 27, 2015, http://www.cancer.org/cancer/ovariancancer/detailedguide/ovarian-cancer-survival-rates.

21. "Acupuncture-Patient Version (PDQ®) Questions and Answers About Acupuncture," National Cancer Institute at the National Institutes of Health, accessed December 28, 2015, http://www.cancer.gov/about-cancer/treatment/cam/patient/acupuncture-pdq/#link/_53.

22. "Paying for Complementary Health Approaches," National Center for Complementary and Integrative Health at the National Institutes of Health, accessed December 28, 2015, https://nccih.nih.gov/health/financial.

23. Barnes et al., "Complementary and Alternative Medicine Use Among Adults and Children."

24. "Prevalence, Cost, and Patterns of CAM Use."

25. M. L. Furlow et al., "Physician and Patient Attitudes Towards Complementary and Alternative Medicine in Obstetrics and Gynecology," *BMC Complementary and Alternative Medicine* 8, no. 35 (2008), doi:10.1186/1472-6882-8-35.

26. "Integration of CAM and Conventional Medicine," in *Complementary and Alternative Medicine in the United States*, Committee on the Use of Complementary and Alternative Medicine by the American Public, Board of Health Promotion and Disease Prevention (Washington, DC: National Academies Press, 2005).

27. L. Dietlind et al., "Physician Attitudes and Knowledge," *eCAM* 3, no. 4 (2006): 495–501.

28. B. R. Greene et al., "Referral Patterns and Attitudes of Primary Care Physicians Towards Chiropractors," *BM Complementary and Alternative Medicine* 6, no. 5 (2006), doi:10.1186/1472-6882-6-5.

29. C. Ritenbaugh et al., "OA16.01. Patients, Physicians, and CAM Providers Regard Communication as Central for Integrating Conventional and CAM Therapies for Chronic Pain," *BMC Complementary and Alternative Medicine* 12, S1 (2012), doi:10.1186/1472-6882-12-S1-O62.

30. "State Map of Current Laws," Center for Nutrition Advocacy, accessed January 5, 2015, http://www.nutritionadvocacy.org/laws-state.

31. Naturopathic Physicians, accessed January 5, 2015, http://www.naturopathic.org.

# 6

# AGING WITH CONTROL

**"M**om, why is it that when babies and kids get older, we call it 'development' but when adults get older we call it 'aging'?"

Whether one is young or old, we are all aging. Progressive changes in appearance, physical abilities, and cognitive performance are a part of the life cycle. However, the vocabulary that you use to differentiate the inevitable changes in children versus adults reflects your cultural perspective on life itself. People celebrate developmental milestones in children but dread them in adults. They are on the perpetual search for the "fountain of youth" and idealize the "prime of life," generally defined as the decade when they are in their forties. But when they reach their sixties, they find that they've become soldiers in a personal war to resist aging. My language may make you uncomfortable, but from the moment of birth, everyone is growing older and in the process of dying.

Getting older is so undesirable in America that it fuels an anti-aging industry worth an estimated $59 billion. As the population continues to live longer, there is an ever-increasing demand for cosmetics, plastic surgery, skin-smoothing injections, nutraceuticals, and sex-boosting hormones.[1] These potions and lotions help mask the physical signs of aging. They also serve a purpose far beyond the concerns of vanity.

Studies show that younger adults in highly industrialized countries have higher societal status.[2] Youth's perceived value is intertwined with the ability to labor and produce; earning power usually diminishes with advancing age.[3] Because earning power is lauded and wisdom and experience are devalued, seniors are marginalized even when they are mentally and physically capable. Superficial physical cues trigger negative age-based stereotypes, so older adults combat ageism by attempting to halt, reverse, or conceal balding, gray hair, wrinkles, and sagging skin. For many older adults, the investment and commitment to cultivating a youthful appearance is a way to continue to be respected and retain opportunities to be relevant.

## Facebook Question

*Julie: My mother is seventy-four years old. Over the last two years, she has steadily become surly. Is it common for the elderly to become more and more negative as time passes?*

*Dr. Georgiou: A mild change in personality can be a normal sign of aging. As people get older, they have fewer filters. But a dramatic shift in personality could be a sign of an underlying medical issue.*

There is a stereotype that older adults are slow, sick, forgetful, hard of hearing, sexless, inflexible, and technologically challenged (among other perceptions).[4] To make matters worse, older people exposed to this prejudice internalize the messages, stereotype themselves, and create a self-fulfilling prophecy. They adapt with negative behaviors, self-deprecating speech (*"I must have had a senior moment."*), and jokes (*"You can't teach an old dog new tricks."*).[5] Then a domino effect ensues. Convinced they are old, individuals develop accelerated physiologic changes that come with age. They may walk more slowly or perform worse on memory testing.[6] Younger adults subconsciously respond by using patronizing elderspeak—slow, loud speech with exaggerated intonation, high pitch, simple grammar, and limited vocabulary. This reinforces the feeling that age has made older adults ineffective at communicating. Over time, their sense of insecurity grows and they may respond with defensiveness and "surly" interactions.

## Archelle's Insider Tips

*Combating ageism with language is an important first step to fostering and achieving the self-respect that is a prerequisite to being respected by others.*

- *Stop—just STOP—making references to your age. Avoid using phrases such as: "senior moment," "gray hair," "halfway to the grave," and "old lady shoes." Others see you as you see yourself.*
- *Don't ignore patronizing speech. Be kind, but assertive.*
- *If someone is speaking loudly, say "You can speak in a normal tone of voice. I can hear you."*
- *If a waiter calls you "dear" or "young lady," extend your hand and say, "My name is Carol. What's yours?"*
- *If the receptionist at your doctor's office says, "Why are we here today?" respond politely with "Well, I am here to follow up on my high blood pressure."*

Ageism makes people feel unimportant and unable to express their priorities, preferences, and choices. These feelings have a significant impact on healthcare decision making.

- Only 21 percent of assisted living residents have primary control of their relocation decisions; for the rest, decisions are made by their children, other family members, friends, and social workers.[7]
- Only 26.3 percent of U.S. adults (and only 33.3 percent of those with a chronic disease) have completed an advance directive and 16.4 percent state that their reason for not completing an advance directive is "my family knows my wishes."[8] Studies repeatedly show that while seniors and their families have many of the same values, they have different perspectives and goals relative to quality of life. As the degree of illness increases, goals become even more divergent.[9]

If you are reading this book, you are someone who wants to feel competent, independent, and in control of the most important aspect of your life—your health. Hopefully that includes being in charge of your health throughout your life, encompassing the journey toward the end of life. The rest of this chapter will show you how to use the CARES model to have a voice in two inevitable decisions: 1) where you live and 2) how you live during the end of life.

## USING CARES FOR DECISIONS AS YOU AGE

Advanced care planning gives you the opportunity to make the best decisions for yourself. This is far preferable to wishful thinking that you can dodge mobility and cognitive issues as well as family conflict associated with end-of-life treatments. Why?

- By age sixty-five, at least one in three adults will have some difficulty with mobility and household activities. By age seventy-five, one in two have difficulty and one in four will need help with bathing, dressing, eating, toileting, getting out of bed, moving around their home, doing laundry, preparing meals, shopping for personal items, paying bills/banking, or handling medications.[10]
- In their final days, nearly a third of older Americans faces critical decisions about whether or not to use life-sustaining interventions, but is unable to participate in those decisions. Too often, conflict ensues. When life-sustaining treatment decisions must be made for patients in the intensive care unit, conflict occurs between the staff and family members in 48 percent of the cases, and between family members in 24 percent.[11]

These statistics exist because thinking about infirmity and the process of dying feels uncomfortable. I get it. As I grow older, the thought of being dependent on and eventually absent from my daughters makes me sad. Some people feel threatened; they believe that talking about death is an omen that kills you. Others believe that planning for death runs counter to their religious beliefs. Conservative Protestants and those with fundamentalist Christian practice are the least likely to plan ahead because they believe that they should not interfere with God's plan for the end of life.[12]

Avoiding conversations that make you think about unpleasant scenarios is a natural and very human response. People have an ingrained, physiologic "fight or flight" reflex that kicks in when they perceive a harmful event, attack, or threat to survival. Running away from the need for advance planning ("I'm too healthy to think about this" or "I don't have time") is simply a protective reflex. However, tactics such as procrastination ("I'll do it later") and denial ("Nothing is going to happen to me") don't change the odds that most people will need some help and all of us will die.

So how do you overcome the innate tendency to flee from age-related conversations and make sure you have a voice even when you can't speak for yourself? I suggest reframing the context of "advance care planning" and "end of life." These terms aren't about dying; they are about living while dying. There is a risk in waiting until a health emergency or crisis occurs to make decisions about senior living arrangements and end-of-life care. If you wait, you—the individual most affected—will have little choice but to passively cede control to family members. Without a plan, you give up the opportunity to develop an approach aligned with your values. Waiting also means that your family will bear the emotional burden of guessing what your preferences might be, the stress of making decisions on your behalf, and potential guilt if they subsequently believe they got it wrong.

## Step 1: Understand Your Condition

People age at different rates. Even within a single individual, organs age differently based on genetic make-up, lifestyle choices, and environmental exposures. The National Institute on Aging explains this beautifully on their website: "At the end of life, each story is different. Death comes suddenly, or a person lingers, gradually failing. For some older people, the body weakens while the mind stays alert. Others remain physically strong, and cognitive losses take a huge toll."[13]

There are a number of credible websites that address the needs of older adults. I use the National Institute on Aging (www.nia.nih.gov) as my "go to" starting point for medical topics and research related to longevity and aging; I surf on AARP's website (www.aarp.org) for lifestyle information.

While it is difficult to accurately predict your specific future needs, this shouldn't be a barrier (or an excuse) from thinking about living arrangements and end of life decisions. In chapter 4, you learned how to use a credible website to educate yourself about the "so what?" of your health condition and the experience you may have in the future. This information is based on the collective experiences of many people who have the same condition. Unless you are a hypochondriac, you know that you will not have every symptom, side effect, or long-term complication. And you may develop a symptom so rare that it isn't listed or even predictable. Nevertheless, the information helped you focus on what to watch for, expect, and guard against in the most likely situations. Similarly, data about the most common health issues and likely circumstances of an aging population can guide you in the planning process. Admittedly, finding the information you need is not so easy.

## Facebook Question

*Harry: My dad had dementia. He died on the first of last month. I want to know if a person can die from dementia?*

*Dr. Georgiou: Harry, I am so sorry for your loss. Dementia is the underlying cause, but not the immediate cause, of death. In dementia, individuals commonly stop eating, which leads to dehydration and low blood pressure. Or, they may forget how to swallow or take a deep breath. When the heart or lungs stop functioning and the brain and organs don't get enough oxygen—cells stop functioning and death occurs.*

Harry's question reflects how hard it is to find a no-nonsense overview of the most common "so what?" issues of aging and end of life. The information is scattered across many different studies and articles. In suggesting that you be proactive about these issues, I realize that it is difficult to even know where to start. To help, I have compiled a Top 10 list of the most common scenarios you are likely to face as you get older.

The first four affect your ability to live independently as you age:

1. You become unable to take care of your basic needs. This includes being able to feed yourself, have bladder and bowel continence, maintain personal grooming and hygiene, walk and move from bed to wheelchair, or perform other daily activities.

    • So what? Consequences range from malnutrition and dehydration to infection and skin breakdown.

2. You can no longer manage your personal responsibilities. These are more complex day-to-day activities and include shopping,

cooking, doing laundry and housework, managing medications and finances, and coordinating transportation.

- So what? Lapses in meeting domestic and financial obligations put your current housing and utilities at risk. The health consequences of missing medical appointments and not filling prescriptions could cause deterioration of chronic health conditions.

3. Your ability to think and interact diminishes. Alzheimer's and dementia are the conditions most often mentioned when discussing older adults' inability to have good judgment and communicate effectively. However, vision and hearing are even more common causes of impairment. National studies indicate that 12 percent of people over sixty-five have moderate or severe vision loss;[14] nearly 25 percent of those aged sixty-five to seventy-four and 50 percent of those who are seventy-five and older have disabling hearing loss.[15]

- So what? Anyone with slow or impaired cognitive ability is vulnerable to physical, emotional, and financial abuse, poor health, and safety issues. Even in the absence of dementia, the consequences of vision and hearing loss should not be underestimated. Hearing and vision loss represent significant safety risks such as falls, unsafe driving, and inability to use a telephone. Vision loss reduces the capacity to read, watch television, or keep personal accounts. Reduced hearing makes it difficult to participate in activities and conversations. The resulting social isolation is associated with a higher risk of death and hospitalization.[16]

4. You experience increasing difficulty with moving and walking. Stiffening joints, arthritis, and reduced flexibility and muscle tone can make moving painful and can increase your risk of falling. Stroke and other illnesses may also present mobility challenges.

- So what? Weakness, instability, and poor balance are the most common threats to your independence.[17] Pets, steps, area rugs, curbs, uneven surfaces, poor lighting, insecure handrails, extension cords, and clutter are a setup for slips, trips, and falls that lead to serious injury, hip fractures, and death.

The next six are the most common issues affecting what happens at the end of life:

5. Your heart stops beating. When the heart stops beating, there is no blood flow, and therefore no oxygen supplying the body's tissues and organs. After approximately four minutes of hypoxia, brain cells start to die. After ten minutes, those brain cells will stop functioning.
6. Your lungs stop breathing. Without lung function, the oxygen in the blood is not replenished, and the consequences are similar to those that occur when the heart stops beating.
7. Your kidneys fail to filter the toxins in your blood. Without the filtering function of healthy kidneys, toxic waste and fluid build up in the body. People can survive with kidney failure for days to weeks, depending on their overall medical condition.
8. Infection invades the bloodstream. Hospitalized patients and those with chronic illness have low immune function and are at higher risk for raging infections. When organisms enter the blood stream, they can multiply in other tissues, causing septic shock and organ failure.
9. Malnutrition results in muscles wasting. When the body's tissues are starved, there are widespread effects ranging from skin breakdown to decreased immunity. One of the most serious consequences is muscle wasting—the body consumes its own muscle mass as a protein and energy source. This affects the respiratory muscles and makes it difficult to breathe.[18]
10. Pain is pervasive and persistent. While not a cause of death, pain affects 46 percent of patients at the end of life. This pain is most often described as bone or joint pain—even by individuals without musculoskeletal disease. The impact of pain on quality of life is significant.

For Step 1, personalize this list. Take your medical conditions into account and add the likely scenarios that you may face. Whether the number of scenarios on your list is ten, twelve, or twenty, writing them down will make this topic less overwhelming as you start to consider your alternatives and preferences.

## Step 2: Know Your Alternatives

There are many options to consider when you address where and how to live as you age. However, decisions are often made with incomplete information. Only 52 percent of Americans who are forty and older are highly confident that they know where to get information about residential alternatives.[19] The medical and legal jargon in living wills is a barrier that prevents many people from understanding their options and communicating their end-of-life care preferences.[20] As with other complex decision-making situations, people resort to the comfort, ease, and simplicity of their biases and perceptions. As long as you are mentally competent, you have a safety net. You can rethink, undo, and redo decisions as often as you want. However, if you become unable to think and interact effectively, you will not have that choice. When you make decisions based on the popular assumptions that I call thought traps, the responsibility for your care will fall to your family and caregivers if you cannot participate in the conversation.

Don't let these common thought traps narrow the choices you deserve to give yourself:

- *"My family will take care of me."* Yes, families are dedicated caregivers. In the United States, there are 31.5 million adults caring for a parent, step-parent, mother-in-law, or father-in-law. And it takes a toll on them. Eleven percent of family caregivers report that caregiving has caused their physical health to deteriorate and 40 to 70 percent of family caregivers have clinically significant symptoms of depression.[21]
- *"I can rely on Medicaid or Medicare for help."* Forty-seven percent of those sixty-five or older believe that Medicare will provide help as they age.[22] The reality is that most long-term care isn't medical care, but rather help with life's everyday activities. While these services (called "custodial care") may keep you safe and prevent the need for medical care, they are not covered by Medicare—at home or in a nursing home—if they are the only help you need.[23]

- *"I can't afford to move into assisted living."* Seventy percent of assisted living residents pay for their living arrangements using personal wealth.[24] But they aren't necessarily wealthy. A variety of financing options such as long-term care insurance, reverse mortgages, or veterans benefits may expand the range of affordable living options.

- *"Moving into assisted living or a nursing home means losing my independence."* Seniors fear losing their independence (26 percent) more than they fear death (3 percent).[25] Yet 93 percent of assisted living residents are satisfied with their level of personal independence.[26]

- *"My family will forget about me in a nursing home."* Studies show that families continue to visit and support their loved ones in residential settings. Nursing home residents get calls or visits from family about forty times a month. The frequency of visits is higher when family lives within a sixty-minute drive of the senior's new residence.[27]

- *"Filling out an advanced directive means they can just pull the plug."* An advance directive states *both* what you want and don't want. Your wishes can go well beyond whether or not you want resuscitation or artificial ventilation. As you will see in a few pages, advance directives enable you to address your medical, emotional, social, and spiritual needs.

Deciding where and how you live as you age is a lifestyle choice that is best made after exploring all your options. Think back to when you bought your first home. Before you even called a realtor, you did your research. What communities are safe? How are the schools? How much could you afford? Even if you had grown up in the area, you took Sunday drives through new neighborhoods to make sure that you'd explored all your options before narrowing your choices. Use AARP.org and the National Institute on Aging websites to research the pros and cons of *all* of your residential and end-of-life treatment options.

The following is a list of the residential options to consider as you age.[28] Keep in mind that the 2016 costs listed will predictably increase by about 4 percent per year.[29]

- *Staying at home or moving in with a caregiver.* Modifications to your home such as adding a front door ramp, installing grab bars in the tub or shower, or converting a first floor den into a bedroom to avoid the stairs may be enough to make home living easier and safer. You can also consider support such as home health and homemaker services. Average cost: $2,400 to $4,800 per month for four to eight hours of services per day. This is in addition to the cost for home modifications.
- *Retirement communities* offer a variety of housing options (apartments, condominiums, detached homes) with social and recreational activities and services geared to seniors. Average cost: highly variable depending on the state and community's real estate market, amenities, and home owner's association dues.
- *Independent living communities* offer a wide range of services such as shuttles, recreation, and laundry service, but typically stop short of providing assistance with basic needs like eating and bathing and personal responsibilities like banking and cooking. "On call" staff are typically available to respond to medical emergencies, but do not provide ongoing care. Average cost: $1,500 to $4,000 per month depending on the state and level of services.[30]
- *Assisted living* offers independent living in an apartment, but with additional support services that are personalized to each resident. Staff are available to assist with a range of services from basic needs to extensive personal assistance. Average cost: $3,600 per month.
- *Memory care* is a type of assisted living that offers specialized assisted living services designed to address the needs of individuals with dementia. Average cost: $5,000 per month.
- *Nursing homes,* also called skilled nursing facilities, offer twenty-four-hour medical care. Residents generally live in private or semiprivate rooms. Average cost: $7,500 per month for a private room.
- *Continuing Care Retirement Communities (CCRC)* offer independent living, assisted living, and nursing home care so that residents can stay in the community even as their needs increase. Average cost: varies widely. Entrance fees guarantee access to a continuum of services "for life" and can start at $20,000 and reach

$1,000,000. Ongoing fees range from $3,000 to $5,000 per month.[31]

Where you live matters. But how you are medically treated at the end of life may matter even more. There are a wide range of options regarding the medical interventions available as you approach the end of life. There are pros and cons to each of these choices. For example, some people feel that a fatal heart rhythm is the best way to die; they want to go quickly and painlessly. Others believe that a sudden death doesn't offer an opportunity to say goodbye to family and friends. With your own priorities in mind, explore each of these options for medical treatment with yourself, your team of advisors, and especially your doctor.

- *Cardiopulmonary resuscitation (CPR)* attempts to restart the heart with an electric shock and chest compressions maintain blood flow until the heart starts beating again. There are no standards for the duration of CPR or the number of times someone can be shocked or defibrillated, but it is well accepted that if the heart is not responding after a reasonable period of time, resuscitation should stop.
- *Ventilators* breathe for you by blowing air into the airways through a breathing tube that is inserted into your windpipe. Because these machines can maintain life for extended periods of time, withholding or withdrawing ventilatory support is one of the most complex and emotional decisions for families and caregivers.
- *Renal dialysis* removes waste from your blood and manages fluid levels if your kidneys no longer function. Dialysis can continue for an indefinite period of time.
- *Antibiotics, antiviral, and antifungal medications* can be used to treat infections.
- *Feeding tubes and intravenous fluids* can be used to address malnutrition and dehydration.
- *Pain medications* can improve quality of life. There are myths that pain medication can accelerate death, but studies show that using narcotics, even high-dose opioids, does not shorten survival at the end of life.[32]

## Step 3: Respect Your Preferences

Your medical condition factors into the alternatives and choices you make, and you can't contemplate alternative living options without also addressing your clinical care needs. However, let me reframe (again) the purpose of planning for your needs as you age: your primary goal is to design a lifestyle—not a cure—that offers the best combination of what you want (your preferences) and what you need.

Nearly 90 percent of people over age sixty-five say they want to remain independent by "aging in place" and staying in their home as long as possible. Eighty percent believe their current home is where they will always live. While this should be possible for most "young-old" seniors who are in their sixties, those in their seventies and eighties will likely need support. Fifty-seven percent of adults who are seventy and older say it's not easy to live independently. Nearly 20 percent need help from caregivers for day-to-day responsibilities. [33]

For Step 3, begin establishing your priorities and preferences by visualizing yourself on a future day. Start with the most common and least threatening scenario—difficulty mobilizing. Imagine that your condition makes it unsafe to remain completely independent in your home. What will your life look like from the moment you wake up until you fall asleep? Be realistic about the challenges and pragmatic about the accommodations as you think about:

- Getting out of bed, bathing, getting dressed, and eating. Who is helping you?
- Doing laundry, grocery shopping, paying bills, and going to the doctor or pharmacy. How are these getting done?
- How you are spending your day? Are you able to read? Use a computer? A telephone? Drive? Are you seeing your friends? Where is your family?

Repeat this exercise as you imagine having difficulty managing your personal responsibilities or performing basic self-care needs. Finally, think about having difficulty interacting with the people around you. Look at the common themes and preferences across these scenarios:

- Environment: Are you staying in your current home, making on-going accommodations, and adding support to address your needs? Or are you downsizing to a more manageable residence where it may be easier to age in place? Alternatively, are you transitioning to a senior living community with more options and amenities for staying physically active?

- Social: Are you maintaining relationships with your current circle of friends? Are you closer or farther from family? Are you in a busy, activity-driven setting or one that is quiet and private?
- Emotional: What is making you smile? What are you accomplishing?

As you think about your living preferences, consider one of the secrets of longevity in the Blue Zones: know why you wake up in the morning. During my visit to Ikaria, I didn't speak to a single older adult who referred to themselves as "retired." Their work was different from what it was in their younger years, but they maintained a strong sense of purpose through their responsibilities. They tended their gardens, cared for grandchildren, or dusted the pews and icons in the village church. As they aged, they didn't retire. They rewired. Know your purpose and design a future home setting that enables you to safely access activities that are rewarding and gratifying. You deserve a future that allows you to continue living a purposeful life for as long as possible.

Respecting your preferences regarding end-of-life decisions revolves around accepting or refusing life-sustaining interventions and technologies. These issues can be distressing to contemplate, which helps explain why many patients "medicalize" their decisions and defer the decision to the healthcare system. Among people who don't have a completed advanced directive, over half are depending on the healthcare system for guidance—40 percent prefer to get information from their doctor and another 13 percent want it from a hospital or healthcare facility.[34]

The scariest thing about death isn't being dead, it's dying. Thoughts about death can trigger fear of the unknown, whereas thoughts about dying bring fear of suffering—physically and emotionally—for yourself and your family. While we can't control death or its mysteries, we can influence our experience to achieve "healthy dying," a term coined by the Tasmanian government in 2011 when the island state launched its Healthy Dying Initiative. Tasmania equates healthy dying to healthy living, reasoning that in both we are engaging actively in the decisions we make.[35] "For the dying person and their family, it means having values and preferences about how and where they receive care at the end of life acknowledged, respected, and supported, and avoiding unnecessary suffering and burdensome treatments."[36]

Healthy living can be easily quantified by measuring blood pressure, body mass index, cholesterol, blood sugar, and other biomarkers. Quantifying "healthy dying" is more challenging. The indicators go beyond physical care decisions to include broader psychosocial goals. Seriously ill patients say that freedom from pain and shortness of breath and anxiety is crucially important. In addition, over 90 percent also refer to a "good death" as an experience where they:

- Are kept clean and maintain their dignity.
- Remain mentally aware and have a sense of humor.
- Have a trusting relationship with their physician and a nurse.
- Know what to expect about their physical condition.
- Have a designated decision maker and someone to talk to about their fears.
- Have their financial affairs in order.
- Have said goodbye to important people.[37]

Healthy dying means flooding your life with experiences that bring you joy and comfort.

Knowing your preferences is critical because your broader priorities are often intertwined with medical treatment decisions. For example, if you want to be mentally aware throughout the dying process, this will influence how your doctor prescribes or administers pain medication and sedatives that diminish your level of consciousness. If you want to be surrounded by friends and family but you also want artificial ventilation discontinued when death is imminent, the timing for discontinuing life support may be postponed to make sure that specific family members or friends are present. While your doctor should be aware of your wishes, you don't need his or her permission to start that discussion with yourself, your family, and those who love you.

To complete Step 3, imagine yourself in a healthy dying experience:

- Personal care and comfort. How do you want to look and feel? What are your preferences regarding bathing, clothing, hair, and grooming? What physical setting will be most comforting to you?

Will you be home? How does the room look? Are there books, music, or pictures that you want within reach?

- Social support. What family or friends do you want close by? How do you want them to interact with you if you can't communicate? Do you want them to pray with you? Do you want visits from clergy or other spiritual support?
- Funeral and memorial plans. Do you want a burial or cremation? What are your preferences regarding organ donation? How do you want to be remembered?
- Medical treatment. Deciding whether you do or don't want resuscitation, artificial ventilation, dialysis, hydration, anti-infectives, hydration, nutrition, and pain medication will vary based on the circumstances. Think through your medical treatment priorities and preferences in the event you are:

  - Critically ill and highly unlikely to survive despite the application of life-sustaining procedures.
  - Permanently unconsciousness.
  - Suffering with an advanced, progressive, incurable condition with complete physical dependency.

- Healthcare agent. Who is the individual you most trust to completely respect your right to get the kind of treatment you want—even if they don't agree with your wishes? Who is best able to handle potential conflict—within the family and with your care providers? Identifying a healthcare agent who can speak on your behalf helps assure that your stated wishes are followed. And because all medical scenarios cannot be foreseen, he or she is also in the best position to understand your goals and make the best decisions for you.

## Step 4: Evaluate Your Options

*"Oh Mom! Don't talk about that stuff! You're too young to talk about dying."* This is how my daughters reacted the first time I started a conversation about my end-of-life wishes. In most families, this avoidance is typical but paradoxical. Ninety percent of people say that talking with family and loved ones about end-of-life care is important, but only

27 percent have actually done so.[38] Why? Because it's hard. Really hard—both for them and for you. But it's easier to have the conversation around a kitchen table than to have this talk in an intensive care unit. If you delay this discussion until there is a healthcare crisis, emotions cloud decision making. If the crisis is serious, you may not be able to participate at all.

After you have arrived at some preliminary decisions about your preferences, it's critical that you share your thoughts and rationale with a team of trusted advisors. These are individuals who you love and trust to have your best interests at heart regarding family, financial, legal, spiritual, and medical issues.

For Step 4, identify your trusted advisors. This may include your:

- Spouse/partner
- Children
- Other family members
- Friends
- Accountant/financial advisor
- Lawyer
- Clergy/spiritual support
- Physician

The work you did earlier in this chapter prepared you to have a thoughtful conversation with your advisors. When you do, remember that *you* are the quarterback of your team. The analogy to football is an apt one. In football, the quarterback has the most difficult job. He determines the strategy, knows all the plays in the playbook, motivates and rallies the team, and ultimately trusts that his teammates will take a ball into the end zone. It all comes together in the huddle where the team gathers in a circle, insulates itself from the noise of the crowd, makes eye-to-eye contact, and connects.

In your conversations, you are the most important player on the team, and the CARES model is your playbook. Your personalized version of the Top 10 list is your offensive move through the aging process; your priorities and preferences for residential and end-of-life treatment alternatives are your defensive strategy. Engaging your team and motivating them to support your decisions means having a huddle with them—not on a playing field, but in a private space without distractions.

Consider gathering your team over a meal when you have this discussion. While satisfying a basic need, food also conveys powerful social meanings—empathy, support, and intimacy. In fact, psychologists have found that sharing a meal makes it easier to talk about stressful or uncomfortable topics.[39]

Archelle's Insider Tip
*There are several online sources that can help you organize and host your huddle, or conversation, with your advisors. My favorites are*

- *Death over Dinner* (http://deathoverdinner.org).
- *The Conversation Project* (http://theconversationproject.org).

*Both offer practical "how to" tools for inviting guests, setting the stage, and jumping into the details of the kind of care you want and don't want for yourself.*

The initial meeting that you have about your aging preferences is simply a kickoff. You and your family may need more than one conversation to work through everyone's feelings, concerns, and ideas. In addition, your kitchen table conversations are not likely to include your doctor, attorney, or accountant. While these advisors are not in a decision-making or authoritative position, their professional recommendations may modify your choices.

Your doctor can help you anticipate some of your specific needs and explain medical treatment options in more detail. Fortunately, as of January 2016, Medicare reimburses doctors for the time they spend discussing advance care planning.[40] This policy change makes it affordable and perfectly acceptable to schedule an office visit specifically for this important discussion. Having a focused discussion about this important chapter of your life is a far preferable option to trying to fit this conversation in during a routine follow-up visit or your annual wellness exam. My recommendation: Do not blur or dilute the purpose of your advance care visit with any other clinical questions.

Your attorneys and estate planner can identify and address potential conflicts among family members, make sure that documents are completed properly, and assure that information is shared appropriately. Your accountant's input may be the most important. He or she can evaluate your future plans and let you know whether your priorities and preferences are financially feasible.

## Step 5: Start Taking Action

The CARES model can help you address your advance care planning, but it is not legally enforceable. An advance directive is a legal document with two parts:

- A living will that documents your preferences for life-sustaining treatments.
- Designation of a durable power of attorney for healthcare. Depending on the state in which you live, this document may also be called a healthcare proxy, medical power of attorney, or appointment of a healthcare agent. The individual you select for this role is a surrogate decision maker if you are incapacitated and the living will does not specify your preferences in a particular medical situation.

There are three key facts to know about advance directives:

- An advance directive can only be completed by you. If you wait too long and become unable to participate in your healthcare decisions, an advance directive cannot be completed on your behalf.
- An advance directive does not take away any of your authority unless you have lost the ability to make decisions for yourself. You always have the right, while you are still competent, to override any preferences you have stated in your directive.
- You can change or revoke advance directives, orally or in writing, at any time and as many times are you want, as long as you remain competent.

For Step 5, you have a greater chance of assuring that your wishes are followed if you have an advance directive. Make sure that all signature lines, witness, and notary requirements are complete. Two additional documents to help assure that your wishes are followed are:

- Durable power of attorney. This document designates an individual to act for you legally if you are incapacitated. You can authorize them to do such things as sign checks and deposit or withdraw funds from your bank accounts. You decide their scope of authority, which can be broad or limited.
- Medical records release. This form gives your doctors permission to share medical records with the individuals you designated as your durable power of attorney for healthcare in your advance directive, your durable power of attorney, and any other family members and friends with whom you want to share information. This is especially important to complete if there is a risk of family conflict and lack of communication.

Too often, important documents, including advance directives, are stashed away in a drawer or safe deposit box and inaccessible to doctors, family, and your power of attorney for healthcare. There's an app for that. Smart phone applications and websites make advance directives easy to access, easy to share, and easy to update online—24/7. The American Bar Association's app, My Health Care Wishes Pro, allows you to store documents on your PDA or tablet. The U.S. Living Will Registry (http://www.uslivingwillregistry.com/howitworksind.shtm) is a service that stores documents in a secure cloud-based database. Everplans (everplans.com) is a comprehensive end-of-life site that allows you to complete and store end-of-life documents as well as information about bank and broker accounts, insurance documents, funeral wishes, social media passwords, and even letters and notes to your family and friends.

My daughters no longer react negatively when I talk about aging. They are used to it. My husband and I have made it an annual winter holiday tradition to review and update our advance directives, wills, and estate plans—followed, of course, by an intimate family lunch with the girls where we discuss the details. Give yourself the life you want and deserve by making your own choices about aging and dying.

## NOTES

1. "Market Overviews: Growth Potential," accessed January 12, 2016, http://www.ageloc.com/content/ageloc/en/anti-aging_trends/market_overviews.html.

2. Corinna E. Löckenhoff et al., "Perceptions of Aging across 26 Cultures and Their Culture-Level Associates," *Psychology and Aging* 24, no. 4 (2009): 941–54.

3. Karina Martinez-Carter, "How the Elderly Are Treated Around the World," *The Week*, July 23, 2013, accessed January 13, 2016.

4. Imogen Lyons, "Public Perceptions of Older People and Ageing," National Center for the Protection of Older People, November 2009, accessed January 14, 2016.

5. Ashley Mae Stripling, "Old Talk: An Examination Of Reports Of Self-Referential And Ageist Speech Across Adulthood," Dissertation Abstract Presented to the Graduate School of the University of Florida in Partial Fulfillment of the Requirements for the Degree Doctorate of Philosophy, August 2011.

6. T. Hess, C. Auman, S. Colcombe, T. Rahhal, "The Impact of Stereotype Threat on Age Differences in Memory Performance," *Journal of Gerontology: Psychological Sciences* 58, no. 1 (2003): P3–P11.

7. Mary Ball et al., "Pathways to Assisted Living," *Journal of Applied Gerontology* 28, no. 1 (February 2009): 81–108.

8. Jaya K. Rao, MD, Lynda A. Anderson, PhD, Feng-Chang Lin, PhD, Jeffrey P. Laux, PhD, "Completion of Advance Directives Among U.S. Consumers," *American Journal of Preventive Medicine* 46, no. 1 (2014): 65–70.

9. K. Kuluski et al., "A Qualitative Descriptive Study on the Alignment of Care Goals between Older Persons with Multi-Morbidities, Their Family Physicians and Informal Caregivers,"*BMC Family Practice* 14 (2013): 133.

10. "Disability and Care Needs of Older Americans: An Analysis of the 2011 National Health and Aging Trends Study," Office of the Assistant Secretary for Planning and Evaluation, April 11, 2014.

11. Catherine M. Breen et al., "Conflict Associated with Decisions to Limit Life-Sustaining Treatment in Intensive Care Units," *Journal of General Internal Medicine* 16, no. 5 (2001): 283–89.

12. Melissa M. Garrido et al., "Pathways from Religion to Advance Care Planning: Beliefs about Control over Length of Life and End-of-Life Values," *The Gerontologist* 53, no. 5 (2013): 801–16.

13. "End of Life: Helping with Comfort and Care," accessed January 28, 2016, https://www.nia.nih.gov/health/publication/end-life-helping-comfort-and-care/introduction.

14. "The State of Vision, Aging, and Public Health in America," CDC's Vision Health Initiative Website, accessed January 27, 2016, http://www.cdc.gov/visionhealth.

15. National Institute on Deafness and Other Communication Disorders (NIDCD), accessed January 27, 2016, http://www.nidcd.nih.gov/health/statistics/pages/quick.aspx.

16. Ann Carrns, "Long-Term Care Costs Rising," *New York Times*, April 9, 2013, accessed April 27, 2016, http://bucks.blogs.nytimes.com/2013/04/09/long-term-care-costs-rising/.

17. "Housing America's Older Adults—Meeting the Needs of an Aging Population," Joint Center for Housing Studies of Harvard University, 2014, accessed January 27, 2016.

18. L. Santarpia, F. Contaldo, F. Pasanisi, "Nutritional Screening and Early Treatment of Malnutrition in Cancer Patients," *Journal of Cachexia, Sarcopenia and Muscle* 2, no. 1 (2077): 27–35.

19. T. Tompson, J. Benz, J. Agiesta, D. Junius, K. Nguyen, and K. Lowell, "Long-term Care: Perceptions, Experiences, and Attitudes among Americans 40 or Older," The Associated Press-NORC Center for Public Affairs Research, April 2013.

20. Lesley S. Castillo et al., "Lost in Translation: The Unintended Consequences of Advance Directive Law on Clinical Care," *Annals of Internal Medicine* 154, no. 2 (2011): 121–28.

21. Family Caregiver Alliance, Selected Caregiver Statistics, accessed February 1, 2016, https://www.caregiver.org/selected-caregiver-statistics.

22. Tompson et al., "Long-term Care."

23. "Long-Term Care," accessed February 1, 2016, https://www.medicare.gov/coverage/long-term-care.html.

24. Assisted Living Facilities, The SBDC National Information Clearinghouse, accessed February 1, 2016, http://www.sbdcnet.org/small-business-research-reports/assisted-living-facilities.

25. Aging in Place in America, Prepared for Clarity by Prince Market Research Final Report, August 20, 2007, accessed February 1, 2016, http://www.slideshare.net/clarityproducts/clarity-2007-aginig-in-place-in-america-2836029.

26. "2013 Survey of Assisted Living Residents," Assisted Living Federation of America, 2013, accessed February 1, 2016, http://www.alfa.org/Document.asp?DocID=512.

27. Cynthia L. Port, Ann L. Gruber-Baldini, Lynda Burton, Mona Baumgarten, J. Richard Hebel, Sheryl Itkin Zimmerman, and Jay Magaziner, "Resident Contact With Family and Friends Following Nursing Home Admission," *The Gerontologist* 41, no. 5 (2001): 589–96.

28. Genworth 2015 Cost of Care Survey, Genworth Financial, 2015, accessed February 1, 2016, https://www.genworth.com/dam/Americas/US/PDFs/Consumer/corporate/130568_040115_gnw.pdf.

29. Ann Carrns, "Long-Term Care Costs Rising," *New York Times*, April 9, 2013, accessed April 27, 2016, http://bucks.blogs.nytimes.com/2013/04/09/long-term-care-costs-rising/.

30. "Independent Living Costs," accessed February 1, 2016, http://www.seniorhomes.com/p/independent-living-costs/.

31. About Continuing Care Retirement Communities, AARP.org, accessed February 1, 2016, http://www.aarp.org/relationships/caregiving-resource-center/info-09-2010/ho_continuing_care_retirement_communities.html.

32. I. Bengoechea, Susana Garcia Gutiérrez, Kalliopi Vrotsou, Miren Josune Onaindia, and Jose Maria Quintana Lopez, "Opioid Use at the End of Life and Survival in a Hospital at Home Unit," *Journal of Palliative Medicine* 13, no. 9 (September 2010): 1079–83.

33. "Inaugural United States of Aging Survey," National Council on Aging, June 2015, accessed February 5, 2016, https://www.ncoa.org/news/press-releases/inaugural-united-states-of/.

34. K. M. Pollack, D. Morhaim, and M. Williams, "The Public's Perspectives on Advance Directives in Maryland: Implications for State Legislative and Regulatory Policy," *Health Policy* 96, no. 1 (2010): 57–63.

35. "Healthy Dying Info Combined," accessed February 8, 2016, http://www.dhhs.tas.gov.au/__data/assets/pdf_file/0006/96378/Web_Healthy_Dying_info_combined.pdf.

36. "An Approach to Healthy Dying in Tasmania: A Policy Framework," Department of Health and Human Services, October 2014, accessed February 8, 2016.

37. K. E. Steinhauser et al., "Factors Considered Important at the End of Life by Patients, Family, Physicians, and Other Care Provider," *The Journal of the American Medical Association* 284 (2000): 2476–82. http://jama.ama-assn.org/content/284/19/2476.full.

38. The Conversation Project, accessed February 10, 2016,http://theconversationproject.org/wp-content/uploads/2015/11/TCP_StarterKit_Final.pdf.

39. M. E. Hamburg, C. Finkenauer, C. Schuengel, "Food for Love: The Role of Food Offering in Empathic Emotion Regulation," *Frontiers in Psychology* 5 (2014): 32.

40. "CMS Finalizes 2016 Medicare Payment Rules for Physicians, Hospitals and Other Providers," CMS Media Release, October 30, 2015, accessed February 15, 2016.

# 7

# SELECTING YOUR HEALTHCARE A-TEAM

**A** future spouse is a lifelong commitment, but a physician's care can have lifelong as well as life-threatening implications. Yet the time people spend getting information about a physician pales in comparison to the time they spend courting and dating a long-term romantic partner. On average, couples date for forty-four months before getting engaged,[1] but Americans only spend 4.6 hours researching the background and credentials of a physician before establishing a relationship.[2] I'm not suggesting that people take three to four years to select a physician, but why don't you commit more time to making an informed decision? Once again, there are unfounded perceptions, or thought traps, that get in the way:

- *"There's not that much difference between physicians."* Unfortunately, all doctors are not created equal. An MD following someone's name does not guarantee consistency or quality. Medical care is not practiced like a recipe, and physicians treating similar patients often come to different conclusions about how to best treat a patient's condition. In addition, physicians have different skill levels. Just as all the players on a baseball team don't have the same batting average, all doctors don't achieve identical outcomes for their patients. Different diagnostic decisions and varying levels of expertise can result in misdiagnosis of conditions, a wide range of infection rates, complications, and even death.

- *"I don't have choice."* Yes, you do. Health insurance companies' list of in-network providers limit, but do not eliminate, your options when choosing doctors. In fact, most states have laws to ensure that provider networks are "adequate." The definition of "adequate" varies in each state, but it rarely means that there is a single doctor in a given specialty. In fact, from a cost perspective, it is in a healthplan's best financial interest to have at least several physicians in each specialty so that the insurer maintains some level of competition and leverage when they negotiate reimbursement rates. Even if you can only choose between two providers, having an option may make the difference between life and death.
- *"I don't think websites with reviews about doctors are valid."* I empathize with this observation because I too have a healthy skepticism about sites that rate doctors solely on patient satisfaction results. Consumers' experiences may be all that's needed to evaluate the quality of hotels and restaurants, but a consumer experience only gives partial insight about the quality of a doctors' care. Patient satisfaction assesses bedside manner and the doctor's office environment, but a friendly bedside manner does not guarantee the quality of a doctor's clinical care. So here's the trap: Consumers' familiarity with opinion-based "Yelp-like" sites for movies, automobiles, travel, and dining reinforces an assumption that consumer opinions are the only source of information available at online physician rating sites. This impression prevents consumers from looking further to identify websites that offer objective information about physicians' professional background and quality of clinical outcomes. Objective sites do exist, and they are free and easy to use. Later in this chapter, I will identify those that I use for credible information.

Consumers primarily consider three factors when selecting a primary care physician:

- Does the physician accept their health insurance?
- Is the office convenient to home or work?[3]
- How quickly can I get an appointment?[4]

This makes sense; primary care is a long-term relationship that needs to be affordable and accessible. But quality considerations are totally absent from these three criteria. During surveys, people say that a physician's malpractice history is an important factor, but 96 percent indicated that they did not check to see if their current primary care physician had any previous claims. Professional qualifications and number of years in practice are also important; however, during the actual process of selecting a physician, only 38 percent of people research the doctors' credentials.[5]

When selecting a surgeon, quality is high on the list of priorities. People report that a surgeon's reputation and competency are *the* most important factors when identifying a doctor for orthopedic, cancer, cardiovascular, and plastic surgery. They want to get "the best" care—in other words, they want to be treated by the doctor with the lowest mortality and morbidity rates. However, people do not select surgeons based on objective performance statistics; they assess competence based on the word-of-mouth recommendations of their referring doctor, family, or friends.[6] For most consumers, the quest for medical quality is merely theoretical—but it doesn't have to be.

Health insurers, federal and state governments, consumer advocacy organizations, and healthcare analytics companies have invested millions to make physician (and hospital) quality data publicly available to consumers. There are over forty websites that provide "report cards" on physicians,[7] but most consumers are unaware of these sites and do not use them. Only 23 percent of Americans have used these sites at all,[8] and only 9 percent have specifically used the quality information from these sites to guide their selection of a doctor.[9]

I've frequently suggested that friends or colleagues use online data to research doctors prior to making a decision about who to see—but few do. They usually come back to me for help and explain that either the information was not what they needed to make a decision or was not presented in a comprehensible way.[10] They don't know how to start or what to look for when selecting a physician. I understand their frustrations; choosing the right doctor is not like choosing a new dishwasher or a new car. There aren't straightforward features and benefits, and you can't rely exclusively on online ratings and reviews. There are a multitude of articles that describe "tips for selecting a physician," but I have not been able to identify a step-by-step process for identifying top candidates and then narrowing the selection down to one physician. Nevertheless, there are over 900,000 actively practicing physicians in the

United States,[11] and you have a responsibility to make an informed decision in selecting the physician who will care for you.

## USING CARES TO SELECT YOUR DOCTOR

You owe it to yourself to identify physicians who will work with you to achieve the best health outcomes, especially when you need surgery and very specialized care. This section gives you the tools to do exactly that.

### Step 1: Understand Your Condition

Facebook Question

> *Michael: I have pain in my knees, thumbs, elbows, and most recently, hips and lower back. Would you visit orthopedics, rheumatology, or family practice?*
>
> *Dr. Georgiou: Start by seeing your primary care physician, either a family practitioner or internist. He or she can evaluate your symptoms and assess whether you have multiple, unrelated joint problems occurring at the same time (like osteoarthritis) or whether you have a single systemic problem that is affecting multiple joints at the same time (like rheumatoid arthritis or lupus). For osteoarthritis, an orthopedist would be the best specialist to see. For rheumatoid arthritis, a rheumatologist would be best. The difference in training and focus in these two specialties is significant.*

Michael's question highlights why identifying the right specialist starts with knowing your diagnosis. If he sees an orthopedist, Michael will likely have a seven-minute interaction with the doctor who will order hand, elbow, back, hip, and knee x-rays followed by an MRI (or two). The orthopedic surgeon is looking for ligament, meniscus, and cartilage problems in the joints, and is ultimately looking for conditions that are treated surgically. A rheumatologist will spend twenty to thirty minutes asking detailed questions about the pattern of joint pain as well as skin, eye, mouth, and gastrointestinal symptoms. While he or she may order one or two x-rays, the more telling diagnostics are extensive (and expensive) blood tests that look for conditions treated with anti-inflammatory medications and immunosuppressants.

A primary care visit doesn't always have to precede seeing a specialist. If you have a long history of migraine headaches with classic but worsening symptoms, you may be confident of your diagnosis and know that you need to see a neurologist specializing in migraine management. However, in other situations, the diagnosis may not be so clear. When a friend with frequent urination asked me to recommend a urologist, I suggested that she see her primary care doctor to narrow down the diagnostic possibilities. Her symptom could be due to a urinary tract infection (easily treated by her primary care physician), pelvic floor weakness (treated by a gynecologist), or an overactive bladder (treated by a urologist).

Being evaluated by the wrong type of specialist has significant clinical and financial implications. Approximately 7.8 percent of all specialist consultations—about 20 million each year—are "clinically inappropriate," meaning that the specialist's training is not the right match for a patient's condition. Sixty-three percent of these patients are re-referred to more suitable physicians, causing wasted time and $1.9 billion in unnecessary copayments. The remaining 37 percent continue to be treated by mismatched specialists,[12] most likely due to specialists' biases. No one, including physicians, is immune to perception errors and thought traps. Specialty physicians are particularly vulnerable to confirmation bias. Their deep knowledge of certain conditions means that they search for and focus on information to confirm diagnoses they know how to treat while ignoring or discounting facts that might steer them into less familiar territory. Surgeons look for opportunities to use steel; cardiologists to place stents; gastroenterologists to insert scopes. This phenomenon is nicely summed up in a quote by psychologist Abraham Maslow, who famously observed, "I suppose it is tempting, if the only tool you have is a hammer, to treat everything as if it were a nail."[13] When it comes to your health, you may need a hammer. Then again, you may need another tool entirely. By taking the time to investigate the most likely diagnosis before you begin looking for a specialist, you put yourself in the best position to find the care you need.

## Step 2: Know Your Alternatives

Facebook Question

> *Earl: I was told by a doctor that my tear ducts are very small and he recommended surgery to enlarge them. Is this risky? Are there side effects? Should I get another opinion?*
>
> *Dr. Georgiou: In adults, tear ducts may become blocked due to thickening of the tear duct lining, nasal or sinus problems, or injuries to the facial bone in that area. If you have excessive tearing or tear duct infections after trying nonsurgical treatments, then tear duct surgery is a reasonable consideration. There are two approaches that can be used, each with different risks. An oculoplastic surgeon is the subspecialist to do this procedure.*

A small tear duct is not a simple problem to correct. The procedure involves cutting a hole into the tear sac, then attaching it to the inside of the nose to improve drainage. Medical and cosmetic complications occur in 10 to 20 percent of cases. Earl was wise to think about getting another opinion regarding his dacryostenosis (dacryo: tear; stenosis: narrowing). However, in addition to wondering "Do I need it?" I hope that my response to Earl prompted him to ask himself "Who should do it?" The goal is to identify a specialist designated as "the best" for your specific diagnosis or procedure. Finding this superstar specialist is not easy.

Earl's eye surgeon is a specialist trained in general ophthalmology. During his training, he probably observed, and maybe even performed, a few of these procedures. However, it is ophthalmologists with subspecialty training in oculoplastic surgery who master the nuanced techniques for performing delicate surgeries on and around the eyelid. And many subspecialists further subspecialize and develop a very niche area of expertise. For example, an oculoplastic surgeon who is a master at endoscopically widening tear ducts is not the same oculoplastic surgeon you'd select for blepharoplasty surgery on drooping eyelids.

These narrow subspecialty areas are not limited to ophthalmology. The top notch neurosurgeon who has removed hundreds of brain tumors is not the surgeon you would select to operate on a herniated cervical disc. A dermatologist who performs hair transplants has different expertise than one who frequently performs Mohs surgery for skin cancer.

Second, while physician-specific outcomes data is collected by all hospitals, it is not available to me, you, most practicing physicians, or your doctor. The information is under lock and key, confidential and protected by the Health Care Quality Improvement Act (HCQIA), which grants legal immunity to physicians and staff who review physician performance.[14] The government's Medicare program also collects this information on physicians, but does not make it publicly available. The result: Physicians are blind to their colleagues' actual quality of care unless they practice together and are in their hospital's elite inner circle. Without access to data, physicians refer patients to specialists based on anecdotes, casual observations, and, yes, their social relationships.

I routinely get calls from family, friends, and friends of friends who want help finding a reputable doctor for conditions ranging from intractable seizures to psoriatic arthritis and uterine fibroids. They call, hoping I might "know someone" or have an "inside track" with quick access to information. I wish I had that inside track, but I don't. I face the same practical barriers as everyone else because the stats on mortality and complications aren't publicly available. However, I have used my CARES model to design a "recipe" that helps identify a narrow list of highly competent specialists. The ingredients are scattered pieces of data, insights and information that *are* available from several different sources. I personally do this research for those who reach out to me. Yes, it takes time, but I get a warm feeling every time a note arrives that says, "Thank you, Archelle. I saw the doctor you recommended, and I feel better knowing that I am in the right hands."

As wonderful as these notes are, they remind me that connecting people to the best healthcare should not be a service limited to those who have my email address or cell phone number. There are many disparities in healthcare. This is one I can do something about. I can show you how to use the CARES model so that you too can make informed choices about the physicians you are going to trust to participate in your care.

To find physicians using this process, you will need online ratings and data. My "go to" website is Healthgrades (www.healthgrades.com). Other sites offer data about providers, but Healthgrades is the most comprehensive. It is a "one-stop" site that includes objective data, satisfaction ratings, and insurance participation information about more than 900,000 doctors and 4,500 hospitals.[15] Bookmark the site so that it's easy to find, and spend time familiarizing yourself with the depth of quality information on the Healthgrades site. For each hospital, there are data on mortality and complication rates for over thirty conditions, patient safety measures, and patient satisfaction reports. For each physician, there are data on educational training, licensure, certification, practice specialty, patient satisfaction, malpractice judgments, and disciplinary actions, as well as the health insurance networks and the hospitals each doctor is affiliated with. Knowing the hospitals where your candidate doctor practices is important—as you will see.

Step 2 begins with identifying the top hospital for your condition—even if you don't anticipate needing inpatient care. As mentioned earlier, doctors' mortality and complication data is not available, but federal law mandates that hospital mortality and complication data be available to the public. Because high-performing hospitals generally attract high-performing doctors, identifying top hospitals for your condition is a gateway to identifying specialists with the best clinical results.

- On the Healthgrades site, search for hospitals in your city and state. The initial search results will include all the hospitals in your area.
- Filter the results by selecting the condition under "Healthgrades Ratings" that is closest to your diagnosis.
- If there is not a perfect match, select a condition within the same organ system. For example, if you have migraine headaches, filter for "Stroke" because they are both neurological conditions.
- If you have a condition that is not similar to any of the condition included under Ratings, filter by "America's Top 100 Hospitals" under Healthgrades Awards.
- From the filtered results, select the hospital with the highest star rating.

Next, call the chief of staff at the hospital you selected. Each hospital has a chief of staff, a physician leader who works with the medical staff, hospital executives, and clinical managers to ensure high-quality care. They are on the "inside track." At minimum, they know who has the most experience—who sees the most patients or performs the highest number of a specific procedure. They also have access to outcomes data collected on physicians and are familiar with physician disciplinary issues. While a chief of staff is prohibited from sharing confidential data, their opinion about the physicians at their hospital is typically well informed.

- Find the name and phone number of the chief of staff on the hospital's website or call the hospital's main information line.
- Contact his or her office. The chief of staff is an actively practicing physician, so keep in mind that most incoming calls are from patients who want to schedule an office visit. Use this script to prevent confusion and communicate clearly with the staff answering your call: *"Hello, this is (your name). I am not Dr. (name)'s patient. I don't need to make an appointment, but I would like to talk with Dr. (name) to discuss a clinical issue related to his/her role as the chief of staff."*
- If Dr. (name) is not available: *"I'd like to leave a message for him or her. Here is my name and number. I'd also be happy to try and reach Dr. (name) again; can you suggest the best time for me to call again?"*
- When you reach the chief of staff, be succinct: *"I have (state your diagnosis). As the chief of staff, I know that you have the best insight about the expertise of the physicians at your hospital."*
- Here are some alternative options to phrase your request: *"I would like to know the doctor you'd most highly recommend for my condition." "If you had this condition, which doctor would you choose to treat you?" "If you have a patient with this condition, who would you send them to?"*

My recommendation to call the chief of staff requires that you have some chutzpah—that's Yiddish for "audacity." I realize that this step is time consuming and it may feel intimidating to you. For hospitals' physician leaders, receiving these calls may feel burdensome. However, because neither hospitals nor the federal government are transparent with physician-specific outcome data, you need to do what it takes to access the best possible care.

Archelle's Insider Tips

- *Do not explain your medical history, review your symptoms, or ask for a referral. The chief of staff is not your physician and does not want to engage in a conversation that establishes a patient-physician relationship.*
- *Do not be satisfied with a recommendation to call the hospital's "referral line." This is merely a marketing service offered by the hospital to their medical staff. Referrals are not based on physician expertise or the quality of outcomes.*

When you have spoken with the chief of staff and obtained a physician recommendation, the hardest step of this process is over. Congratulations.

Next, tap into the "wisdom of the many." Your primary care physician may have suggested a specialist for your care. Or your specialist may have recommended a subspecialist. However, in the absence of data, these recommendations are merely an opinion. Any one opinion, even that of a highly educated professional, is not as valuable as the aggregate opinion of a larger group of diverse individuals. This concept of "the wisdom of the many" is as old as Aristotle,[16] and people tap into this philosophy when accessing reviews for cars, professors, or home contractors.

- Reach out to people within your social network who have had a health situation similar to yours. Ask:

  - What condition the specialist treated and/or what procedure was performed.
  - How *they* initially identified that specialist.
  - Whether they would go back to that specialist.

- Caution: Do not react to specialists' names or attempt to validate names already on your list by asking, "Have you ever heard of Dr. (name)?" Peer pressure is powerful. People tend to respond to the information you give them. You don't want to limit your contacts' responses by mentioning a name you've already gathered. You are looking for untarnished and independent opinions.

Finally, narrow the list of physician names recommended by the chief of staff, your primary care physician, and your social network by identifying the handful of specialists whose names are repeatedly mentioned. This short list represents the collective wisdom of the group and prepares you for the next step.

## Step 3: Respect Your Preferences

In 1987, President Ronald Reagan said, "Trust but verify." This signature quote referred to onsite inspections confirming the commitments of the United States and Russia to reduce their nuclear arms. Verifying the information provided in a negotiation can further promote trust between two parties and, most importantly, help prevent a disaster later.

A poignant story from my days in private practice illustrates why Reagan's advice also applies to healthcare. In the early 1990s, an experienced obstetrician-gynecologist relocated to northern California and set up her practice in our medical community. Her beautiful new office, complete with granite countertops and fresh flowers, and her wholesome Midwest personality were an appealing draw for patients needing gynecological care. Several of my patients were first-time pregnant mothers; they raved about this doctor's kind and supportive maternal bedside manner. I trusted my patients' reviews, but I didn't independently verify this doctor's clinical expertise. If I'd spoken to colleagues in her specialty, I might have been privy to the hushed hallway conversations about the series of babies she'd injured during forceps deliveries and I might have been told about the women whose routine gynecological procedures resulted in serious bladder and ureter complications. I referred a stream of patients to this doctor until the competency issues became public, triggering a state medical board investigation. Unfortunately, the investigation occurred only after one baby had a disastrous result.

Verifying information has come a long way since 1992, when my best option was word-of-mouth information about my colleague's skills and practice patterns. Today, online research about this same obstetrician-gynecologist quickly shows that the Medical Board of California suspended her license for "repeated negligent acts" and put her on probation for five years. She relocated her practice back to the Midwest, where her license was *again* suspended by that state's medical board after another series of complications. As I write, this physician continues to do surgery and deliver babies for unsuspecting patients. Why? Currently, she has resolved the issues in the state where she practices and has an unrestricted medical license. Unless her patients take the time to research her history, they will probably remain unaware of her suspensions and probations.

The reality is that no one is obliged to warn you about another physician's experience or competence. You can trust, but the responsibility rests with you to verify. When I review a physician profile, I focus on specialty board certification, practice specialization, disciplinary actions, and medical malpractice history. This information is publicly available and at your fingertips. None of these individual indicators is a definitive measure of quality, but collectively they are a barometer of the level of care and expertise you can expect. Along with information about office location, the insurance plans accepted, and patient satisfaction ratings, you have data at your fingertips that can help you navigate toward the best physician for you.

For Step 3, I have outlined the profile indicators I check when researching a physician. They are listed in priority order, assuring that quality always trumps convenience. All the information you need is available on Healthgrades.com. There you can create side-by-side comparisons of any doctor in the country.

- Board certification: If a physician is board certified, this means that he or she has completed a minimum of two additional years of full-time specialty training *after* finishing medical school and one year of internship. More importantly, he or she has passed tests to assure that they have the knowledge, experience, and skills for a particular specialty. Not board certified? Take it as a warning. It suggests that a physician didn't get additional training or didn't pass the certification tests. Even if a physician is board certified, don't go to the next step before making sure the certification is in the specialty you need. For example, if you are researching a rheumatologist, your candidate may be board certified by the American Board of Internal Medicine, but you also want to verify that they have subspecialty certification by the American Board of Rheumatology. If you have an irregular heart rhythm

that requires electrical mapping and an implantable cardiac defib-
rillator, a board-certified cardiologist should also be certified in
cardiac electrophysiology.

Exclude physicians who are not board certified. Don't worry. There are
about 690,000 board certified physicians in the United States.[17] Of
those 690,000 physicians, 229,000 of them are certified in a subspecialty.[18] In other words, there are ample highly qualified physicians to
choose from.

Archelle's Insider Tip

*Where a physician went to medical school is irrelevant. Why? Medi-
cal school admission is based primarily on undergraduate grade point
average and scores on medical school entrance exams. By the time a
physician is practicing, both of those indicators are over five years old,
and neither correlates with a doctor's quality of care.*

- Practice specialization: Even when doctors are board certified in a
  specialty or subspecialty, they can have a clinical focus *within
  their specialty*. For example, all gastroenterologists perform colo-
  noscopies to screen for colon cancer, but some further specialize
  in treating specific conditions such as inflammatory bowel disease
  (Crohn's disease and ulcerative colitis), liver disease, or gastroe-
  sophageal reflux (heartburn). Doctors who see a higher than average number of patients with a specific condition have greater
  experience and therefore better outcomes because "practice
  makes (almost) perfect." Yes, that's intuitive, but since 1979,
  multiple published scientific studies confirm that the volume of
  procedures a doctor performs correlates with the quality of his or
  her results.[19] For example, the risk of dying after having aortic
  valve replacement surgery was 6.5 percent among heart surgeons
  who perform a high volume of heart surgeries. Among surgeons
  performing a low volume of heart surgeries, the risk of death rises
  to 9.1 percent.[20] The risk of complications after low back surgery
  was 27 percent lower when the surgery was performed by a high
  versus a very low volume surgeon.[21] Don't be complacent. Even
  for more routine surgeries, such as laparoscopic hysterectomy, the
  volume of surgeries your doctor performs matters. Low-volume

gynecologists have a higher rate of failed procedures that require converting to an open abdominal hysterectomy compared to high-volume gynecologists.[22]

Physicians with the highest "Experience Match" score on their Health-grades profile are those who see the highest volume of patients with specific conditions and/or perform the highest volume of procedures. Use this score to further narrow your list of physicians. Keep in mind that a difference of two to three points in the Experience Score is not significant, but larger differences do matter. They reflect a meaningful difference in level of expertise.

Archelle's Insider Tip

*Healthgrades uses software technology to generate the Experience Score and does not disclose the exact volume of patients or procedures. If you are selecting a general surgeon (for gall bladder removal), urologist (for prostate removal), orthopedist (for knee or hip replacement surgery), or a spine surgeon (for cervical or lumbar spine surgery), you can get more specific information on the number of surgeries performed (along with complication and mortality rates) by going to ProPublica's Surgeon Scorecard (https://www.propublica.org/data/).*

- Malpractice history: Seventy-five percent of physicians will be sued sometime during their careers,[23] therefore a single malpractice case in a doctor's profile is difficult to interpret. Multiple cases, however, are reason to pause. Check to see if the physicians you are considering have malpractice judgments in their profile. Here's how to interpret the data you find:

  - If there are no malpractice judgments: Don't allow yourself to have a false sense of reassurance. Ninety-seven percent of cases settle out of court, and most state medical boards only disclose information about payments made for court-recorded medical malpractice judgments.[24] For these reasons, information on the vast majority of cases is not available.
  - If there is one judgment: This may be a signal that a physician has poor bedside manner, but doesn't necessarily reflect the quality of their outcomes. Review their patient satisfaction ratings to get insight to their communication

skills and relationships with patients. Doctors with the lowest patient satisfaction ratings have twice as many malpractice suits.[25]

- If there are two or more malpractice judgments: Think twice about establishing a relationship. Multiple judgments may signal a quality-of-care issue.

- Disciplinary action: Punitive actions by medical licensing boards are uncommon because states are obliged to offer due process prior to sanctioning a physician's license. This expensive legal process means that states limit their investigations to physicians with the most egregious behaviors; consequently only about 0.3 percent of physicians—about 2,700 in the entire United States—are disciplined each year.[26] Boards rarely suspend or revoke physicians' licenses because of the devastating career impact. The most common disciplinary actions are public reprimands, probation, and fines. The majority of these physicians continue practicing without an obligation to proactively share this information with patients or colleagues. Unless you look for this information, you may never know that your doctor has a troubled professional history.

Similar to malpractice suits, a clean record does not offer conclusive insight about the quality of a doctor's practice. However, the presence of a single disciplinary action in a physician's profile suggests serious professional conduct issues. My uncategorical recommendation is to stop considering a physician with a medical board blemish. Why such a harsh stance? There may be additional worrisome behaviors that are not publicly disclosed. Don't take the risk.

- Patient satisfaction: Satisfaction ratings are influenced by communication, ease of getting an appointment, and waiting times, as well as the physical qualities of the facility. They reflect consumer perceptions of the doctor and office staff. High ratings *are* correlated with doctors who have better interpersonal skills and offer more health education to patients.[27] Important? Absolutely, but there is no correlation between a pleasant demeanor and better clinical outcomes. Use satisfaction ratings to break a tie if quality-of-care indicators (board certification, practice specialization, malpractice history, and disciplinary actions) are equal.

If you've followed the process, the one physician whose name remains on your list meets the CARES checklist of objective quality criteria.

## Step 4: Evaluate Your Options

You've completed the necessary steps to "trust but verify." This final step in your evaluation represents the art of combining data with your personal priorities and preferences. In this step, you focus on how you *feel* when interacting with this physician.

### Facebook Question

*Cheryl: I have a very athletic thirteen-year-old boy who was recently diagnosed with hip dysplasia. We have been to two orthopedic surgeons, and they each recommended different procedures. The pediatric orthopedist recommended a hip replacement. We are tempted to get a third opinion on what should be done. What are your thoughts?*

*Dr. Georgiou: I applaud you for getting two opinions and, if you are not feeling comfortable (which is probably why you are writing to me), then you should absolutely get a third. But don't get just any third opinion. Make sure that you see a surgeon with a lot of experience in caring for teenagers with hip dysplasia. As you know, in a young person with hip dysplasia, the acetabulum (the hip socket) has not developed properly and is too shallow to fit the ball of the femur (the thigh bone). Since an adolescent is still growing, the ideal treatment preserves the natural hip bones for as long as possible, sometimes through surgery that restores the normal anatomy of the joint. Hip replacement surgery, which involves putting in a prosthetic metal hip, is rarely a good option for thirteen-year-olds since it puts them at risk for a lifetime of orthopedic complications. I don't know what your son needs since I am not an orthopedic surgeon, but I do know that you need an opinion that you trust.*

As a mother, Cheryl's question had a dramatic impact on me. I could feel her fear emanating from the screen of my computer while I was reading her post. She was responsible for selecting the surgeon, and the choice of surgeon dictated the surgery. Making the wrong decision could affect her son's ability to walk normally for the rest of his life. She didn't know where to turn, and because I hadn't published this book, I couldn't share the CARES model and my process for selecting the right physician. So I decided to go beyond my usual arm's length relationship with viewers. I asked Cheryl to contact me on my private email. After asking a few more questions about her son, Preston, I offered to do the research to find the nation's experts in treating adolescents with hip dysplasia. Within forty-eight hours, I got back to Cheryl with the names of three nationally renowned surgeons. Coincidentally, one was in Minneapolis.

Cheryl jumped on the information and scheduled an appointment with the Minneapolis specialist. I had suggested that she refer to the visit as a "consultation" rather than a "second opinion" (or in her case, a third opinion). The American Medical Association uses these terms interchangeably, but for physicians, and especially for surgeons, the language you use influences their behavior.

- A "second opinion" visit translates to: "Tell me if my first doctor was right." A physician's responsibility is to agree or disagree with the diagnosis and treatment plan laid out by the first physician. As a result, the visit is focused on and biased by the original diagnosis and treatment plan. If both physicians are practicing in the same medical community, he or she may agree with the first opinion (as long as it's not blatantly wrong) to avoid contradicting the judgment of a colleague.
- A "consultation" translates to: "Tell me what's wrong and the best way to treat it." A physician feels responsible for offering an independent expert assessment of your medical condition. He or she considers previous diagnoses, but otherwise starts with a fresh, clean slate and offers his or her best thinking and unfiltered recommendation.

Immediately after the consultation with this Minneapolis physician, Cheryl was confident she had identified "the best" doctor for Preston.

Highly competent? Absolutely. He had successfully treated many teens with hip dysplasia by doing surgery that would reshape, but not damage, the joint. Although his credentials were impeccable, it was the partnership she *felt* with this doctor that reassured her. He laid out all the options, answered questions, and drew sketches to explain what would happen in the operating room. Then when they started to discuss the recovery process, he asked Cheryl questions and solicited her expertise as a parent. He wanted her input regarding the physical therapy regimen, the style of wheelchair, how and when Preston could get back to school, and when Preston would potentially resume his athletic activities. Four months later, Cheryl sent me a picture of Preston shooting hoops on the basketball court. A year later, I featured Cheryl and Preston on a special news segment and interviewed them about the importance of getting a second or third "consultation."

Figuring out whether you and a physician can have an effective partnership regarding your health is a conclusion you can reach *only after* having a face-to-face interaction. There is no obligation to continue seeing a physician simply because you had an initial visit. Unfortunately, people tend to commit to being treated by a physician at the moment they walk into the office, rather than waiting until the end of the visit, when they can assess whether or not there's good chemistry. This "I'm here . . . I might as well" approach may be an efficient way to get treatment for a minor, routine problem, but it's not a smart shortcut when selecting a doctor. Imagine buying a car without test driving it. Over 80 percent of prospective car owners do their online homework on a vehicle's gas mileage, interior space, trunk capacity, and safety before they show up at the dealership. However, 84 percent also take the car out for a test drive before making a purchase. Sitting in the driver's seat is the only way to feel the comfort and the smoothness of the ride, how the car handles a sharp turn, and the responsiveness to quick steering wheel adjustments.[28] Similarly, conversing in the exam room is the only way to test your comfort with a physician and the care they deliver.

For Step 4, schedule a consultation with the highly credentialed physician you identified. Be prepared to focus on more than just the medical recommendations. Pay attention to whether the communication and interaction during the visit has the characteristics of a collaborative patient-physician relationship. Here are some factors for you to consider:

- Do you feel comfortable asking questions—even about topics not raised by the physician?
- Does the physician answer questions using words and phrases that you understand?
- Do you feel comfortable admitting your fears and expressing your preferences?
- Does the physician listen and respond to your concerns?
- Do you feel comfortable disagreeing with a point of view or recommendation?
- Does the physician try to call all the shots? Do you? There shouldn't be a power battle.

You deserve a physician that encourages and expects you to be an active participant in your care. If you feel unsure, intimidated, disempowered, or have more questions after your visit than before it started—listen to your intuition. Resist the "I might as well" mindset. If there is a recommendation to schedule surgery or an invasive procedure, simply say, "I need to think about it." Then schedule a consultation with another highly qualified specialist from your original list and get another opinion. This process may sound time intensive, but there is no substitute if you are committed to finding the best care. Remember, Cheryl needed three "test drives" to find the best physician for Preston.

## Step 5: Start Taking Action

Taking action means knowing "what's next?" in your newly established relationship with a physician. It also means taking personal responsibility for getting all your medical records to your new doctor, rather than assuming that your doctors will share information with each other. Here's why: In 1996, the federal government passed the Health Insurance Portability and Accountability Act (HIPAA) to protect the confidentiality of patients' medical information. Unfortunately, even when you sign a records release form, the law makes it burdensome for physicians to share your medical information with each other. Electronic health records add further complexity. Despite the federal government's $35 billion investment in electronic health record systems for doctors and hospitals, these systems are not wired to talk to each other.[29] Each doctor's office manages its own electronic fortress of information, and the only practical way to share records is old-fashioned printing and mailing.

When your records are incomplete, there can be unintended consequences. You might experience delays in treatment (to wait for records to arrive), diagnostic errors (due to lack of medical history and context), and duplication of tests that were already performed (if the previous results are not accessible). I've seen compelling examples of these consequences in my husband's practice. As a gastroenterologist, David frequently consults with new patients who travel to the Twin Cities from rural Minnesota communities with complaints of persistent abdominal pain, gas, and bloating. About one-third of the patients arrive with incomplete medical records. Depending on the urgency and level of concern, David may repeat some blood tests. Occasionally, he will repeat a colonoscopy because it is faster to redo the procedure than to try to track down the results of a previous procedure.[30]

As a patient, you have the right to access and obtain copies of any health information in doctor, provider, or healthplan records. And you can duplicate and share any of your medical information with anyone, *without* the bureaucracy of HIPAA. The fastest, cheapest, and most efficient way to assure that every doctor has access to all your records is to give them a comprehensive set yourself.

For Step 5, start by collecting copies of all your historical records dating back three to five years. Then on an ongoing basis, and with every single visit, get copies of new:

- Laboratory test results,
- Radiology reports,
- EKGs and other diagnostic tests,
- Specialty consultation summaries,
- And operative reports, including results of surgical pathology.

No matter how brilliant, experienced, or empathetic your physician may be, his or her effectiveness ultimately depends on your commitment to staying actively engaged. You and your physician are in a relationship that is committed to your health, and relationships are, by definition, interdependent.

## NOTES

1. "Women Are Dating Longer Before Getting Engaged," *BrideBox.com*, accessed February 23, 2016, http://www.bridebox.com/blog/couples-date-before-engagement.

2. Healthgrades Consumer Survey, *Healthgrades.com*, accessed proprietary data 2012, http://www.healthgrades.com/.

3. D. A. Hanauer et al., "Public Awareness, Perception, and Use of Online Physician Rating Sites," *The Journal of the American Medical Association* 311, no. 7 (2014): 734–35.

4. Ibid.

5. E. Sonny Butler, "Consumers Ranking of Criteria for Selection of a Primary Care Physician, 2002," *International Association for Computer Information Systems*, accessed February 25, 2016, http://iacis.org/iis/2002/ButlerMcGlone.pdf.

6. Alexander T. Yahanda et al., "A Systematic Review of the Factors that Patients Use to Choose Their Surgeon," *World Journal of Surgery* 40, no. 1 (January 2016): 45–55.

7. Sabriya Rice, "Dealing with Online Ratings Often Proves Challenging for Doctors," *Modern Healthcare* (March 1, 2014), accessed online February 25, 2016, http://www.modernhealthcare.com/article/20140301/MAGAZINE/303019970.

8. Hanauer et al., "Public Awareness, Perception, and Use of Online Physician Rating Sites."

9. Tamara Rosin, "Consumers Value Objectivity over Accuracy When Seeking Medical Information: 8 Findings," Becker's Hospital Review, November 17, 2014, accessed February 25, 2016, http://www.beckershospitalreview.com/hospital-physician-relationships/consumers-value-objectivity-over-accuracy-when-seeking-medical-information-8-findings.html.

10. Hanauer et al., "Public Awareness, Perception, and Use of Online Physician Rating Sites."

11. "Total Professionally Active Physicians," Kaiser Family Foundation, January 2016, accessed February 24, 2016, http://kff.org/other/state-indicator/total-active-physicians/.

12. "2014 Physician Referral Survey," Kyrrus, 2014, accessed March 1, 2016, https://www.kyruus.com/hubfs/Kyrruus_Whitepaper_Physician_

Referral_Sentiment.pdf?submissionGuid=2366d71e-30d9-4811-bdd8-df1118df813b.

13. Abraham Maslow, "Acquiring Knowledge of a Person as a Task for the Scientist," in *The Psychology of Science: A Reconnaissance* (Chapel Hill, NC: Maurice Bassett Publishing, 2007), 15, https://books.google.com/books?id=3_40fK8PW6QC&q=hammer#v=snippet&q=hammer&f=false.

14. D. Vyas and A. E. Hozain, "Clinical Peer Review in the United States: History, Legal Development and Subsequent Abuse," *World Journal of Gastroenterology* 20, no. 21 (June 7, 2014): 6357–63, doi:10.3748/wjg.v20.i21.6357.

15. "Healthgrades 2016 Report to the Nation," *Healthgrades*, October 2015, accessed March 4, 2016, http://www.healthgrades.com/quality/healthgrades-2016-report-to-the-nation.

16. Josiah Ober, "An Aristotelian Middle Way Between Deliberation and Independent-Guess Aggregation" (Stanford/Princeton Working Papers, September 2009), accessed March 8, 2016, https://www.princeton.edu/~pswpc/pdfs/ober/090901.pdf.

17. *U.S. Medical Regulatory Trends and Actions* (Federation of State Medical Boards, May 2014), accessed March 20, 2016, https://www.fsmb.org/Media/Default/PDF/FSMB/Publications/us_medical_regulatory_trends_actions.pdf.

18. *2013–2014 ABMS Board Certification Report* (American Board of Medical Specialties, 2015), accessed March 20, 2016, http://www.abmsdirectory.com/pdf/Resources_certification_statistics.pdf.

19. H. S. Luft et al., "Should Operations Be Regionalized? The Empirical Relation Between Surgical Volume and Mortality," *The New England Journal of Medicine* 301, no. 25 (1979): 1364–69.

20. John D. Birkmeyer, MD, et al., "Surgeon Volume and Operative Mortality in the United States," *The New England Journal of Medicine* 349 (November 27, 2003): 2117–27, doi:10.1056/NEJMsa035205.

21. H. H. Dasenbrock et al., "The Impact of Provider Volume on the Outcomes After Surgery for Lumbar Spinal Stenosis," *Neurosurgery* 70, no. 6 (June 2012): 1346–54, doi:10.1227/NEU.0b013e318251791a.

22. R. H. Andries et al., "Clinical Relevance of Conversion Rate and Its Evaluation in Laparoscopic Hysterectomy," *Journal of Minimally Invasive Gynecology* 20, no. 1 (January–February 2013): 64–72.

23. A. B. Jena et al., "Malpractice Risk According to Physician Specialty," *The New England Journal of Medicine* 365, no. 7 (2011): 629–36.

24. "Medical Malpractice Basics," *Medical Malpractice*, accessed March 18, 2016, http://www.medicalmalpractice.com/topics/medical-malpractice-basics.

25.  Henry Thomas Stelfox, MD, PhD, et al., "The Relation of Patient Satisfaction with Complaints Against Physicians and Malpractice Lawsuits," *The American Journal of Medicine* 118, no. 10 (October 2005): 1126–33.

26.  Sidney M. Wolfe, MD, et al., "Public Citizen's Health Research Group Ranking of the Rate of State Medical Boards' Serious Disciplinary Actions, 2009-2011," *Public Citizen*, May 17, 2012, accessed March 20, 2016, http://www.citizen.org/documents/2034.pdf.

27.  C. Laine et al., "Important Elements of Outpatient Care: A Comparison of Patients' and Physicians' Opinions," *Annals of Internal Medicine* 125, no. 8 (October 15, 1996): 640–45.

28.  "New Research: One in Six Car Buyers Skips Test-Drive; Nearly Half Visit Just One (Or No) Dealership Prior to Purchase," *PR Newswire*, April 15, 2014, accessed March 25, 2016, http://www.prnewswire.com/news-releases/new-research-1-in-6-car-buyers-skips-test-drive-nearly-half-visit-just-one-or-no-dealership-prior-to-purchase-255302891.html.

29.  "Where Is Hitech's $35 Billion Dollar Investment Going?" *Health Affairs Blog*, accessed March 28, 2016, http://healthaffairs.org/blog/2015/03/04/where-is-hitechs-35-billion-dollar-investment-going/.

30.  Personal interview with Dr. David Feldshon, March 28, 2016.

# 8

# POWER SHOPPING FOR HEALTH INSURANCE

**B**uying health insurance is confusing. Paying for insurance is expensive. Using it is complex. No wonder nearly two-thirds of Americans say shopping for health insurance is as bad as having a tooth filled and 73 percent say that deciphering the complexities of insurance is worse than being stuffed into the middle seat on an airplane.[1]

Arielle, my oldest daughter, experienced this frustration when she turned twenty-six and could no longer be covered by our health insurance policy. As a full-time law student, she didn't have the option of getting a policy through an employer, so I suggested she "go shopping" on the New York health insurance exchange established by the Affordable Care Act. Wanting her to take responsibility, I offered to help—but only after she did some research and narrowed down her buying choices. When the enrollment deadline was a few days away, she called me, somewhat exasperated. "Mom, I don't know where to start. I don't know what I need. I don't know what's important. There are too many options and it's overwhelming. Can you just tell me what to do?" Arielle was certainly capable of using the Web to purchase health insurance, but she wanted to make an informed decision and purchase the *right* insurance plan with the *best* coverage at the *best* price for her.

Selecting a policy was not intuitive or easy for Arielle, even with the advantages of a college education and a mother who was a managed care executive. Imagine how hard it was for the other 7.2 million people who were first-time buyers of health insurance in 2014 and 2015[2] and how hard it will be for the 40 million people who will buy their own insurance by 2018.[3] On average, consumers have to sort through the nuances of thirty different healthplan options offered by five different insurance companies before making a choice.[4] Among the 147 million people getting insurance through an employer, the range of options is smaller, but picking the best plan can still be a hand-wringing experience.

For Arielle, the annual premiums for an individual policy ranged from $5,300 to $9,000. For a family policy, the average annual premium was $16,800.[5] This is equivalent to buying a small economy car—every single year. However, while 79 percent of car owners are satisfied with their vehicle purchase, consumer satisfaction with health insurance is at 69 percent—the lowest rating in the last ten years and in the bottom five of all industry satisfaction rates tracked by the American Customer Satisfaction Index.[6] Even fewer consumers, 49 percent, trust their health insurer.[7] As an industry insider, I have witnessed the lack of transparency, bureaucracy, and poor customer service that prompts consumers to question the integrity of the health insurance industry. However, I have also seen how consumers, or healthplan enrollees, are themselves responsible for some of the negative perceptions.

The Kaiser Family Foundation conducted a survey asking adults ten questions to gauge their knowledge of how health insurance works. Only 57 percent knew what a provider network was and only 51 percent could correctly calculate the out-of-pocket cost for a hospital stay.[8] Most people could not imagine buying a new car without knowing what features are included in the price, yet a study published in the *Journal of Health Economics* showed that only one in seven Americans understands the basic components of a health insurance plan.[9] Nevertheless, each year they sign up for health insurance without knowing what they're getting or what they can expect. Too often, they default to "I hope my insurance covers the bills." This self-imposed unpredictability erodes trust and creates stress because deductibles, copayments, coinsurance, and payment policies can translate into substantial annual out-of-pocket costs.

## USING CARES TO BUY HEALTH INSURANCE

Here's the good news: The basics of health insurance are straightforward and easy to understand when explained in plain English rather than legalese. And as long as you can do some simple math, you can estimate the financial impact of all your plan options. This chapter shows you how to use the CARES model to select the right coverage before you make this large annual investment.

### Step 1: Understand Your Condition

Between 2011 and 2016, health insurance premiums increased 20 percent and deductibles increased 63 percent.[10] As politicians and the media tout the industry's profits and scrutinize executives' lavish salaries, insurers are often seen as the villains responsible for escalating costs. But they aren't. Here's why: As medical costs increase, health insurance costs increase proportionately. And insurance companies can only stay afloat if they collect more money than they pay out to reimburse providers—doctors, hospitals, home care providers, pharmacies, and equipment suppliers—for the care they deliver. In 2010, Americans spent an average of $7,428 per person on medical care; in 2015, they spent $10,742.[11] That's a 45 percent increase that, not surprisingly, parallels the insurance increases during that same period of time. While you may not personally spend this much, there are others who have extraordinarily high medical costs. Insurers set prices based on the "community average" cost, which spreads that cost and financial risk across the population. At some point in the future, the individual with extraordinary medical costs could be you.

Facebook Question

*Jim: Why buy insurance at all? Wouldn't it work better to put money aside, build up the funds, and pay as you go?*

*Dr. Georgiou: Your idea is a good one, theoretically, but the reality is that most of us don't have enough savings to cover the cost of a serious medical problem. Did you know that unpaid medical bills are the leading cause of bankruptcy in the United States? That's why it's important for every individual to have health insurance. Unfortunately, even people with insurance accumulate medical bills they can't pay off because they can't afford the out-of-pocket costs.*

There are many factors that cause medical costs to continually increase—aging, technology, new medications, and consumers' demand for care. While you can't control the total cost of the population you are pooled in, you do have some control over the cost of your own care. How? You can influence the pace of your financial outlay for health insurance and medical care through your choice of plan design—the combinations of premium, deductibles, copayments, coinsurance, and other out-of-pocket costs.

Selecting the best plan design starts with anticipating your upcoming care needs and predicting how much you will likely incur in medical bills next year. In Step 1, the focus is estimating your future medical visits and care events so that you can calculate the amount you are likely to spend next year.

1. Predictable events. You can anticipate many of the healthcare visits you will have next year. Look ahead and list the number of:

- Office visits for preventive care and follow-ups for chronic conditions and ongoing medical issues. (For example, do you have a yearly follow-up visit to discuss your blood pressure and medication? Does your doctor have you come back twice yearly in order to refill your antidepressant medication?)
- Laboratory tests, radiology exams, and other procedures to monitor your current condition. (For example, does your cardiologist order an annual EKG or echocardiogram? Do you have regular blood tests to monitor your blood sugar and cholesterol?)
- Inpatient (hospital) or outpatient (surgery center) admissions for planned medical or surgical care. (For example, are you pregnant or planning to get pregnant? Are you finally going to get your shoulder repaired? Do your pacemaker batteries need to be replaced?)
- Home healthcare visits, physical therapy sessions, medical devices, or equipment for recovery from elective medical or surgical care.

List each visit, procedure, test, or admission in a separate row on a lined sheet of paper or a spreadsheet. If you are purchasing insurance for your family, be sure to organize the information so that you can easily identify which family member will receive each service. This is important because insurance policies set different amounts for individual and family deductibles and out-of-pocket maximums.

2. Potential events: There isn't a crystal ball to foresee new medical problems that may develop, but many people have patterns regarding how often they access acute, urgent, or emergent care services. (For example, do you inevitably have one migraine a year that requires injectable pain medication for relief at an urgent care? Does at least one of your children end up in the emergency room each year with a sprain, fracture, or a big cut that needs stitches? Do you typically see your doctor one or two extra times a year for a cold, back pain, a urinary tract infection, abdominal pain, or a rash?) Look at how you used healthcare and your insurance over the last two years. Make some realistic assumptions about the number of visits in the upcoming year. Include the number of:

- Office visits to primary care doctors or specialists.
- Urgent care visits.
- Emergency room visits.
- Add these potential encounters to your list.

3. Estimate the cost for each predictable and potential medical encounter. It is extremely difficult to know exactly how much future visits or events will cost because prices for healthcare services vary significantly among providers, contract rates vary by insurance company, and the complexity of your situation influences how much is charged. However, online tools can help you estimate the cost of each encounter and arm you with enough data to analyze your healthplan options. Don't be tempted to abandon this step because the data is not perfect; using reasonable estimates is a better alternative than making a decision based on no data at all.

If you have health insurance, your healthplan may offer a "healthcare cost estimator" that lists average prices for services based on their contracted rates with in-network providers. Alternatively, my preferred site for getting this information is Healthcare Bluebook (healthcare-bluebook.com). The site is free and publishes a "fair price" for various medical services based on the typical fee that providers in your area accept as payment from insurance companies.[12] Bookmark this site. If you have unanticipated medical needs, it will also help you predict what your medical bills may amount to well before you receive the "balance due" from your providers.

4. Estimate next year's total medical costs. Total the costs for all the predictable and potential healthcare services you are likely to have in the upcoming year. This reflects how much, at a minimum, you are going to use your insurance. You'll use this total when you Evaluate Your Options later in the chapter.

### Step 2: Know Your Alternatives

For most consumers selecting insurance, the top priority is picking a plan with the lowest cost.[13] Unfortunately, too many people don't know the basics of insurance and define "lowest cost" as the plan with the lowest premium or lowest deductible. This is short-sighted. It doesn't take into account how copayments, coinsurance, out-of-pocket maximums, and out-of-network coverage contribute to total out-of-pocket costs. Insurers capitalize on consumers' naïveté by "shrouding"—selectively displaying features of the plan and hiding the negative add-on costs built into the plan design. However, shrouding only works when consumers are myopic about their choices.[14] The next section will keep you from being blindsided. I'll define the key terms you need to know and build a hypothetical scenario to show you how each feature affects your out-of-pocket costs.

*Premium:* The amount you pay for insurance during a policy year. Your annual health insurance premium is a sunk cost. You pay it whether you receive care or not. This cost should be factored into your personal budget.

Scenario: Assume your monthly premium is $500. Over the course of the year, you will pay $6,000 = $500 x 12 months.

*Deductible:* The amount you contribute toward your medical costs *before* your insurance company pays for any benefits during a policy year. Don't avoid high deductible plans if you are healthy. Your out-of-pocket costs will be lower if you select a plan with a high deductible and low premium because you *only* have to pay toward the deductible if you receive care. Note: The Affordable Care Act regulations mandate that preventive services (like immunizations and screening tests) are not subject to the deductible and are paid at 100 percent. Your insurance will pay for these services even before you meet the deductible.

Scenario: Assume your deductible is $1,500. You see your primary care doctor for abdominal pain. The visit, x-rays, and blood tests add up to a total of $500. If you have not had any previous medical services during the year, then you must pay the entire $500 bill. You will have to pay an additional $1,000 out of pocket for any future services before your insurance will pay for any of your care. Here is a summary of your insurance costs and coverage so far:

Your cumulative contribution for medical care: $500

The cumulative contribution paid by your insurance company: $0

*Copayment:* A specified dollar amount you contribute toward the cost of a service. Copayments for primary care visits may be lower than specialist visits, and there may be specific copayments for emergency room, urgent care, and hospital admissions. A copayment counts toward your annual deductible amount. Don't get seduced by low copayments. Copayments *only apply* after you meet the deductible.

Scenario: Assume your emergency room visit copayment is $100. You have an ER visit for nausea and vomiting, and the bill totals $2,000 in total allowed charges. Because you've already paid $500 toward your deductible, you must pay $1,000: $100 copayment for the ER visit plus an additional $900 to meet the deductible. Your insurance company pays the remaining $1,000 balance.

Your cumulative contribution for medical care: $500 + $1000 = $1,500

The cumulative contribution paid by your insurance company: $0 + $1,000

*Coinsurance:* A specified percentage you contribute toward the cost of a specific service. The financial impact of coinsurance adds up quickly, yet one-third of consumers do not understand how to calculate these costs.[15] Coinsurance is frequently stated as a fraction, 80/20 or 70/30, to show the cost-sharing split between you and your insurer. The higher number is usually the insurer's portion of the responsibility; the lower number is yours.

Scenario: Assume you have a 20 percent coinsurance for inpatient admissions. After your ER visit, a surgeon determines you need to be hospitalized for gallbladder surgery. The hospital charges are $5,000. Because you've met your deductible, you pay 20 percent of $5,000 = $1,000, and your insurance pays $4,000.

Your cumulative contribution for medical care: $1,500 + $1,000 = $2,500

The cumulative contribution paid by your insurance company: $1,000 + $4,000 = $5,000

*Out-of-Pocket Maximum:* The most you'll have to contribute toward the cost of your medical care during a policy year. After meeting the out-of-pocket maximum, all medical expenses are covered 100 percent. Deductibles, copayments, and coinsurance accumulate toward the out-of-pocket maximum, but premiums do not. Hopefully, you will never need so much care that you reach your out-of-pocket maximum, but this amount of money should be earmarked in your savings—just in case you need it.

Scenario: Assume you have a $7,500 out-of-pocket maximum. You have a serious infection after your surgery and need to be readmitted. The inpatient medical bill is $50,000. The 20 percent coinsurance would make you responsible for 20 percent, or $10,000. However, because you've already paid $2,500 (in deductibles, copayments, and coinsurance), then you are only responsible for paying $5,000 to reach the out-of-pocket maximum. Your insurance will pay the remaining $45,000 balance.

Your cumulative contribution for medical care: $2,500 + $5,000 = $7,500

The cumulative contribution paid by your insurance company: $5,000 + $45,000 = $50,000

*Out-of-Network Benefit:* A specified percentage of the allowed amount that your insurance will pay for care from out-of-network providers.

Make sure you fully understand your coverage for out-of-network care. Selecting the best plan design starts with anticipating your upcoming care needs and predicting how much you will likely incur in medical bills from doctors and other providers who are not in your network— not contracted with your insurance company.

This is the least transparent aspect of plan design and can create the most financial vulnerability. Make sure you know the difference between your provider's charges and your insurer's "allowed charges." The "allowed" amount is the reimbursement that your insurer believes is a fair rate for a specific service. It is inevitably much less than providers charge, and an out-of-network provider has no obligation to accept this rate as the full payment. You are responsible for the entire balance. There are two additional points to remember.

- The amount you pay toward out-of-network care may not count toward your deductible or your out-of-pocket maximum. Many plan designs have a separate, substantially higher, out-of-network deductible and out-of-pocket maximum that you must reach before your insurance pays 100 percent.
- You are responsible for knowing the network status for all the providers who are involved in your care. Just because your doctor refers you to a radiologist, a physical therapist, or a laboratory doesn't assure that you are being treated by a contracted provider.

While you may be willing to pay the out-of-network balance, make an informed decision rather than being shocked by a whopping balance after you have received care. Insurance companies do not publish allowed amounts or make them readily available, but they will give you this information if you or the out-of-network provider call the health-plan's customer service line with specific procedure and diagnosis codes.

Scenario: Assume you have a 70 percent out-of-network benefit. You decide to have a prominent orthopedic surgeon repair a shoulder injury that's been bothering you for years. The orthopedist is out of network and his charge for surgery is $15,000. However, the insurance company's allowed amount for this procedure is $8,000. Your insurance will pay 70 percent of $8,000 = $5,600. Your out of pocket is the entire balance: $15,000 − $5,600 = $9,400. Ouch!

Your cumulative contribution for medical care: $7,500 + $9,400 = $16,900

The cumulative contribution paid by your insurance company: $50,000 + $5,600 = $55,600

If you add your annual premium cost ($6,000) to your cumulative contribution for medical care, your *actual* total, the amount you'll pay for insurance and medical care, is: $16,900 + $6,000 = $24,900. While this seems like an extraordinary amount of money to pay, remember that without insurance you would be responsible for 100 percent of the medical costs. In this scenario, that's $72,500.

Understanding these six basic terms (premium, deductible, copayment, coinsurance, out-of-pocket maximum, and out-of-network benefit) will get you well on your way to being literate in the language of health insurance. This literacy is critical to making better decisions when you buy insurance, and it is also the knowledge you need to advocate for yourself. Unless you know the language of health insurance, you cannot effectively communicate with your insurer about what they paid, and more importantly, what they denied.

## Step 3: Respect Your Preferences

*Every* purchase has trade-offs. The lower monthly payments of a five-year car loan feel more affordable compared to those in a three-year loan even though the cumulative amount of interest is significantly higher. Sport tires offer high-precision handling but a bumpier ride than touring tires. Larger cars are more comfortable but less fuel efficient. Even with services as essential as health insurance, you can't have it all.

For insurers, the cost of their policies must be affordable while at the same time being sufficiently high to cover the total cost of the medical care (or else the insurance company will go out of business). So insurers design policies that allow consumers to make trade-offs in four categories: financial risk, choice, access, and coverage. Knowing your preferences helps assure that you make the right decisions and that you are aware of trade-offs *in advance* rather than when you are in the midst of a medical situation. In the next section of this chapter, I'll explain each of the four trade-offs you need to understand.

Remember, healthplans shroud information. They show you what they *want* you to know rather than what you *need* to know to make an informed decision. Therefore creating your own summary of each healthplan's features will allow you to compare your options side by side and ensures that you know what you will really be signing up for.

*Financial Risk*: Selecting health insurance includes some degree of gambling. More than 44 percent of Americans prefer lower premiums and a higher deductible. They like lower sunk cost (premium payments) in exchange for "rolling the dice" on the deductible. If they need unexpected medical care, they'll have to pay more before their insurance kicks in. But if they stay healthy, they're ahead financially. On the other hand, 36 percent of Americans want a lower deductible, even if it means paying a higher monthly payment.[16] They accept higher upfront costs for the peace of mind they get from having lower unpredictable out-of-pocket exposure. These vastly different preferences are based on individuals' varying comfort levels with accepting financial risk regarding their medical costs. The premium trade-off is straightforward:

- A lower monthly premium always means that the combined cost of deductibles, copayments, co-insurance, and out-of-pocket maximums is higher.
- A higher monthly premium means that the combined cost of deductibles, copayments, coinsurance, and out-of-pocket maximums is lower.

For Step 3, create a chart with a column for each healthplan option, and a row for each of four trade-offs: financial risk, choice, access, and coverage. List the premium, deductible, copayment, coinsurance, out-of-pocket maximum, and out-of-network benefit for each plan option.

## Archelle's Insider Tip

*Don't be fooled. You have not hit the jackpot if you find an insurance plan that has both a low premium and a low deductible. Heath insurers hire smart mathematicians, and there will inevitably be another feature—usually a sky-high coinsurance—that allows the insurer to make up the difference.*

*Choice:* Providers who contract with insurers accept lower reimbursement rates in exchange for being listed as "in-network" and having easier access to the insurer's patients. For consumers, large, inclusive networks are appealing. Having more choice in your plan means there's less chance of needing to switch doctors to stay in-network or being told that "the best" doctor is not accessible. However, plans that offer more choice are more expensive because insurers have less negotiating power, particularly with popular specialists and prestigious, brand name hospitals. Higher reimbursement rates mean higher medical costs, which get passed along to you, the consumer, through higher premiums, deductibles, copayments, and coinsurance.

Insurers pressure hospitals and doctors to accept low rates; those who don't are simply excluded from the network altogether. The premiums for narrow-network plans can be 5 to 20 percent cheaper.[17] But there can be significant consumer dissatisfaction. Some patients don't realize the restrictiveness of the network until they need specialized medical care; others find out that a hospital or doctor is out-of-network only after they get an unexpected high bill for the out-of-network balance.

Expand the information in your chart by checking and indicating the network status of certain key providers:

- Your primary care physician.
- Any specialists you see on a regular basis.
- The university hospital or academic medical center in your city.
- If you have children, the children's specialty hospital.

Archelle's Insider Tip

*Narrow network plans do not have a "WARNING" sign to cue you in to the limited choices before you enroll. All plans are simply required to have directories that list the providers who are contracted, and it's up to you to decide whether a plan's network is too narrow for you.*

*Access:* Primary care physicians (PCPs) are generalists. They focus on preventive care and address straightforward medical problems. When deciding on the best next steps for complex conditions or persistent symptoms, PCPs, unlike specialists, are not narrowly focused on a single organ system. This lack of bias combined with their clinical skills allows them to direct patients toward the right type of specialist and avoid unnecessary specialist visits that may occur when patients self-refer. While there are valid clinical reasons to establish a solid relationship with a PCP, many healthplans *require* that patients coordinate all care through PCPs who act as "gatekeepers" to specialists. This is an insurance company strategy to decrease overall medical costs because requiring a PCP referral before receiving specialty care decreases overall insurer costs by about 6 percent.[18] This savings is passed along to consumers in the form of lower premiums and deductibles.

Your trade-off for a slightly lower cost is tolerating the inconvenience and bureaucracy of a gatekeeper model. Imagine that you have recurrent actinic keratoses, precancerous skin lesions typically caused by many years of sun exposure. You recognize the characteristic lesions, and there is no question they must be removed because 10 percent turn into squamous cell skin cancer. In a nongatekeeper "open access" model, you can self-refer to a dermatologist. In a gatekeeper model, you must incur the inconvenience of a PCP visit even though you know that you need a referral. There are countless scenarios in which direct access to specialist care from the inception of a condition is more cost-effective, but in a gatekeeper model, you have to follow the rules or risk having coverage for your specialist visit denied.

Continue to expand your chart. For each healthplan option, indicate whether there is a gatekeeper model or open access for specialist referrals.

### Archelle's Insider Tip

*Healthplans offering "open access" plans will promote this feature because it is appealing to consumers. However, "open access" only refers to in-network specialists. Some plans have zero coverage for care by out-of-network specialists.*

*Coverage:* Benefit coverage refers to the specific medical services that a health insurance policy includes and excludes—in other words, what the insurer pays for and doesn't pay for. This is the most difficult trade-off category to clarify and quantify because even though the Affordable Care Act requires that all benefit plans cover ten essential benefits, insurers have leeway in how they interpret their coverage obligation. Making this even more complicated, insurers can have their own proprietary interpretation guidelines that are not published in the documents that you receive when you enroll. So even if you read your policy cover to cover, you will not know all the coverage rules they can impose to say "no." Here are two examples.

## Facebook Question

*Jackie: My husband has had kidney stones for many years. He probably passes one a week. He has tried diet change but a nutritionist might be able to help. Are nutritionist visits covered under insurance plans?*

*Dr. Georgiou: Jackie, depending on the chemical analysis of his stones, there may be dietary changes that can decrease stone formation. However, all insurance benefit plan designs are different. To find out whether they will cover nutritionist visits, call the customer service number on the back of your husband's insurance card.*

I couldn't answer Jackie's simple question because there is not a single answer. Since the passage of the Affordable Care Act, all plans cover outpatient services, which includes nutrition/dietary counseling, but:

- Some plans only cover in-network dieticians, not nutritionists.
- Some plans limit coverage to patients with end-stage renal (kidney) failure. Having kidney stones does not qualify for coverage.
- The number of visits varies by plan. Some pay for six annual visits, others for ten.

## Facebook Question

*Ellie: Do insurance companies pay for the breast cancer gene test or is it out of pocket? Is it expensive?*

*Dr. Georgiou: Most insurance companies will cover the cost of BRCA1 and BRCA2 testing (the genetic tests for hereditary breast cancer) for individuals who have either a personal history or family history of certain cancers. If you pay out of pocket, the cost of these tests can range from several hundred to several thousand dollars.*

The answer is "it depends"—again. All plans cover laboratory services; however, most only cover BRCA testing when there is a high risk of *hereditary* breast cancer. For Ellie, the tests will be reimbursed if she meets her healthplan's high-risk criteria, but not if she is merely curious or concerned about her genetic status. This seems straightforward unless you ask, "When is someone considered high risk for hereditary breast cancer?" It varies. Each healthplan has medical directors, and the criteria are based on their individual interpretation of published medical studies.

Benefit coverage criteria are not transparent and the decisions are steeped in clinical nuance. It might be tempting to ignore this trade-off until you need care and then cross your fingers that your medical situation meets the coverage criteria so that your bills are paid. Instead, I recommend that you familiarize yourself with the most commonly misunderstood benefit coverage issues and do some due diligence for specific benefits that may be relevant to you.

The document that gives you this information is called the Evidence of Coverage (EOC). This is the binding legal contract that describes the healthcare benefits covered by the healthplan and is much more detailed than the snapshot of information on the website or the Summary Plan Description (SPD) that is posted online or included in your enrollment materials. Many healthplans have their EOC online, but they bury it on their website and force you to navigate through multiple links to find it. Because healthplans are required to file their EOCs with the state, it's easier find this document through a Google search. Use the following format: "Evidence of Coverage for (Insurance Company) (Name of Plan Design)" (for example, "Evidence of Coverage for Care 1st AdvantageOptimum Plan HMO").

Obtain the Evidence of Coverage for each plan option you are considering. You don't have to read this document in its entirety. Focus on the following sections.

- Exclusions: This section is one of the most important in the entire document. It outlines all the medical services that are not covered under any circumstances or only when specific criteria are present. Read the entire section.
- Use the EOC's table of contents or the "Find" function on your computer to find the details on:

- Physical, speech, and occupational therapy: These services are covered but frequently only as long as the treatment is restorative, meaning as long as an individual continues to make progress. This requirement limits coverage for individuals with chronic disabilities (cerebral palsy, spinal cord injury, multiple sclerosis, stroke) who benefit from therapy but don't make functional improvements.
- Chiropractic care: Some plans completely exclude coverage for chiropractic care. Others exclude it unless the chiropractor is treating a spinal condition.
- Bariatric (obesity) surgery: Some plans have a blanket exclusion for bariatric surgery. Others cover bariatric surgery for morbid obesity. This means that an individual's body mass index must be over forty.
- Infertility services: Coverage for infertility varies significantly from plan to plan. There may be no coverage at all, coverage only for diagnostic testing, or coverage for services including in vitro fertilization.
- Hearing services: Hearing tests are covered by the majority of plans, but coverage for hearing aids varies. Some plans have a blanket exclusion, while others offer a dollar allowance toward the purchase price of a hearing device every two to three years.

To complete Step 3, identify the exclusions and limitations categories that matter to you, and make sure you fully understand each plan's coverage. If the language in a plan's EOC is vague, call the customer service phone number to get clarification. Include coverage information on your chart.

### Archelle's Insider Tips

*If you are trying to figure out whether an insurance document is the Evidence of Coverage or the Summary Plan Description, look at the number of pages. An EOC has seventy to one hundred pages. An SPD has fifteen to twenty pages.*

*The EOC for every plan states that services covered must be "medically necessary." On the surface, this seems reasonable. Unfortunately, what this really means is that the healthplan's medical director, not your doctor, makes the final determination regarding the medical necessity of any surgery, procedure, lab test, or medical service. Insurers are required to reconsider their decision when patients file an appeal; the process is included in the EOC under "Appeals."*

## Step 4: Evaluate Your Options

This chapter has focused on the financial implications of health insurance options—frankly because they are easy to define and quantify. However, studies show that consumers' most important goal when buying insurance is having peace of mind.[19] For some, this means having a low deductible even if a high-deductible plan makes more economic sense. For others, sleeping soundly at night means having generous out-of-network coverage so that there are no financial boundaries to keep preferred doctors and hospitals from being accessible. The emotional aspects of the selection process are subjective and sometimes irrational, nevertheless these aspects are equally important to address—as long as you are informed.

Throughout the previous sections, you've been using the CARES model to assemble a significant amount of information.

- Your predicted medical care needs and costs for the upcoming year (Understand Your Condition).
- The six basic financial details for each plan option you are considering (Know Your Alternatives).
- The trade-offs for each plan (Respect Your Preferences).

Step 4 begins with calculating the actual financial differences between each plan option. With those facts, you can decide how willing and able you are to take financial risk. Last but not least, you must be honest with yourself about the nonfinancial trade-offs you can tolerate.

Here is how to do the math.

For each plan option, enter:

a. Plan monthly premium
b. Plan deductible
c. Plan copayment amounts
d. Plan coinsurance percentage (the lower percentage)
e. Maximum out-of-pocket costs

f. Next year's total medical cost from Step 1 (Understand Your Condition)

Then calculate:

g. Annual premium (multiply a x 12)
h. Amount of the deductible that you will pay (insert b or f, whichever is less)
i. Medical costs that exceed your deductible (subtract f – b)
j. Amount of copayments that you will pay*

  * Add together the copayments you'll pay for each visit/encounter

k. Amount of coinsurance that you will pay (multiply d x i)
l. Your cumulative contribution for medical care (add h + j + k)*

  * If the cumulative contribution is more than your maximum out-of-pocket costs (e), replace l with the amount in e because this is the maximum out-of-pocket cost you pay in a premium year.

m. Your TOTAL* cost (add g to l)

  * This combines your cumulative contribution and the insurance premium.

I used this worksheet approach to evaluate three different plans for Samantha, a healthy twenty-eight-year-old whose medical needs included seeing a primary care physician for preventive care, a gynecologist for contraception, and a neurologist for Botox® injections for migraine headaches four times a year. The total costs per plan ranged from $8,900 to $10,200 to $17,800. The cost differences between the three options were mind-boggling, and she was tempted to select the cheapest plan until I explained the trade-offs:

- The least expensive plan was a gatekeeper plan with a narrow network and no out-of-network benefit.
- The intermediate cost plan was open access for specialist referrals, included a broader network of providers, but had no out-of-network benefit.
- The most expensive plan was an open access plan with the same broad network of providers as the intermediate plan, along with 70 percent out-of-network benefit coverage.

Samantha selected the intermediate cost plan. While her total costs would be at least $1,300 more than the least expensive plan, she wanted the convenience of being able to bypass her primary care physician when it was time for her neurology appointments. She also got peace of mind knowing that the most prominent hospital in her city was in-network.

## Step 5: Start Taking Action

Most individuals make their healthplan selections in the fall. In December or early January, the new insurance card along with a thick folder of information arrives in the mail. How many times have you put the new card in your wallet and tossed the folder in a drawer? I am guilty of that myself, so I won't suggest that you read these materials cover to cover.

However, for Step 5, I strongly suggest that you at least read the Summary Plan Description (SPD) that summarizes the key features of the policy. Focus on:

- What's covered.
- What's excluded.
- Your contribution toward the cost of medical services you receive: deductible, copayments, coinsurance, out-of-pocket maximum, and out-of-network benefits.
- The plan's requirements for specialist referrals and prior authorization for hospitalizations and other services.
- Your appeal and grievance rights.

There is no Hippocratic oath written into your insurance policy because health insurance is not healthcare; it is a merely a financial contract between you and the insurer. However, it may be the most important contract you ever sign because it makes healthcare affordable, accessible, and can prevent you from having a financial crisis. Know how it works. Know the rules. Know your rights. Know your obligations. Make yourself as familiar with your policy as you are with a new car: know how to take advantage of all the features while staying safe. And remember, a new car salesman doesn't expect you to read the manufacturer's automobile manual; he or she makes sure you know it's in the glove compartment in case you have a malfunction. Similarly, you don't have to read the entire Evidence of Coverage, but you should make sure that it is quickly accessible if you need to refer to it.

## NOTES

1. Jay MacDonald, "How Bad Is Shopping for Health Insurance?" *Bankrate.com*, accessed April 12, 2016, http://www.bankrate.com/finance/insurance/health-insurance-poll-1114.aspx#ixzz45ftVhpJH.

2. "ObamaCare Facts: Facts on the Affordable Care Act," Obamacare Facts, accessed April 4, 2016, http://obamacarefacts.com/obamacare-facts/.

3. "Accenture Consulting Research Report, 2014," *Accenture Consulting*, accessed April 4, 2016, https://www.accenture.com/us-en/insight-private-health-insurance-exchange-annual-enrollment.aspx.

4. Reflects 2017 statistics and data from the states on the Federal Exchange.

5. "Health Insurance: Premiums and Increases," National Conference of State Legislatures, accessed April 5, 2015, http://www.ncsl.org/research/health/health-insurance-premiums.aspx.

6. "Benchmarks by Industry," American Customer Satisfaction Index, accessed April 5, 2015, http://www.theacsi.org/customer-satisfaction-benchmarks/benchmarks-by-industry.

7. PARTNERS+simons, "Partners+Simons National Healthcare Trust Index Shows Five Times More Americans Trust Their Health Plan Than Congress," news release, October 12, 2015, accessed April 5, 2015, http://www.marketwired.com/press-release/partnerssimons-national-healthcare-trust-index-shows-five-times-more-americans-trust-2062985.htm.

8. Mira Norton et al., "Accessing Americans' Familiarity with Health Insurance Terms and Concepts," *KFF.org*, November 11, 2014, http://kff.org/health-reform/poll-finding/assessing-americans-familiarity-with-health-insurance-terms-and-concepts/.

9. George Lowenstein et al., "Consumers' Misunderstanding of Health Insurance," *Journal of Health Economics* 32, no. 5 (September 2013): 850–62.

10. "2016 Employer Health Benefits Survey," Kaiser Family Foundation, September 14, 2016, accessed November 11, 2016, http://kff.org/health-costs/report/2016-employer-health-benefits-survey/.

11. Calculated from data in "Medical Cost Trend: Behind the Numbers 2016," PwC Health Research Institute and "NHE Fact Sheet," CMS.gov, accessed April 8, 2016, https://www.cms.gov/research-statistics-data-and-systems/statistics-trends-and-reports/nationalhealthexpenddata/nhe-fact-sheet.html.

12. Healthcare Bluebook, accessed April 9, 2016, https://healthcareblue-book.com.

13. "The New Era of Narrow Networks: Do They Come at the Cost of Quality?" *Health Affairs Blog*, October 13, 2015, accessed April 9, 2015, http://healthaffairs.org/blog/2015/10/13/the-new-era-of-narrow-networks-do-they-come-at-the-cost-of-quality/.

14. Xavier Gabaix and David Laibson, "Shrouded Attributes, Consumer Myopia, and Information Suppression In Competitive Markets," National Bureau of Economic Research, November 2005, accessed April 10, 2016, http://www.nber.org/papers/w11755.pdf.

15. Lowenstein et al., "Consumers' Misunderstanding of Health Insurance."

16. MacDonald, "How Bad Is Shopping for Health Insurance?"

17. "Milliman Report: High-Value Healthcare Provider Networks," America's Health Insurance Plans, July 1, 2014, accessed April 15, 2014, https://ahip.org/wp-content/uploads/2016/02/High-Value-Provider-Networks-Issue-Paper-2014_07_01.final-pdf.pdf.

18. Based on analysis of 2007–2011 data in "HMO vs PPO," *Diffen.com*, accessed April 16, 2015, http://www.diffen.com/difference/HMO_vs_PPO.

19. Jenny A. Cordina et al., "The Role of Emotions in Buying Health Insurance," *McKinsey&Company*, accessed April 19, 2016, http://health-care.mckinsey.com/sites/default/files/768912_The_role_of_emotions_in_buying_health_insurance.pdf.

# 9

# USING CARES EVERY DAY

I've shown you how to use the CARES model to make complex healthcare decisions. Investing the time to do your own research, answer questions, and complete activities informs you about your condition, alternatives, and preferences before making important choices. However, using the model isn't limited to serious or life-threatening situations. And all health issues don't require an extensive analysis. You can use the basic components of the model to help you answer your own questions and make smart choices for the common healthcare dilemmas you face every day.

When I answer questions on Facebook or email, I naturally think through the basic elements of the CARES model before I craft my answers. I've done it so many times, it's almost reflexive. Just as I use "go to" websites, I use the model's "go to" questions:

- Understand Your Condition: So what?
- Know Your Alternatives: What else?
- Respect Your Preferences: What matters most?
- Evaluate Your Options: What gives you peace of mind?
- Start Taking Action: What's next?

Some questions take me just one or two minutes to research and answer; others require a little more time. Admittedly, my medical expertise accelerates the process. However, if you become familiar with the model and use it regularly, you will find yourself becoming more self-reliant with your own health.

In this chapter I will share a series of viewers' questions and my brief online responses. My goal is to show you how these viewers could have answered their question using the CARES model quickly, easily, and independently. Keep in mind that these examples are intended to demonstrate how to use the model; they are not a textbook of medical details for the clinical scenarios. And in some cases, I've made assumptions about the viewer's circumstances in order to show you how to make this model work for you at home.

Facebook Question

*Jen: There is no doubt in my mind that my husband has sleep apnea. I talk to him about having it diagnosed, but all he comes up with is "What will they do to treat it?" Could you tell me some examples of how apnea may be treated?*

*Dr. Georgiou: Sleep apnea is a serious issue and if your husband knows the complications, he may be more willing to address it. The underlying problem with sleep apnea is that his body, his heart, and his brain are not getting enough oxygen while he is sleeping. There are multiple treatments available including face masks that force air into the airway to keep it open and dental devices. Occasionally surgery is necessary.*

While her question focused on treatments, the issue making Jen's husband resistant to being evaluated was not understanding the dangers associated with sleep apnea. A common misperception is that sleep apnea is no different than snoring or simply a form of insomnia. The first step for Jen was influencing her husband to get care.

Jen could use the "Understand Your Condition" portion of the CARES model to understand the "so what?" and "why bother?" of sleep apnea—and then share it with her husband.

- "Go to" MayoClinic.org.
- Link to the Patient Care and Health Information section and search "sleep apnea."
- Read the Definition to understand the physical abnormality causing sleep apnea, then read about the complications for a summary of the wide-ranging medical side effects that include type 2 di-

abetes, high blood pressure, risk of heart attack, and liver problems.

- The Treatment section lists an array of interventions, from airway masks to surgery.

## Facebook Question

*Angie: I have rotator cuff syndrome. Is surgery necessary? I just began physical therapy.*

*Dr. Georgiou: Conservative treatments such as rest, ice, and physical therapy often are all that's needed to recover from a rotator cuff injury. Injuries involving a complete tear of the muscle or tendon may need surgical repair.*

Rotator cuff syndrome is one of the most common causes of shoulder pain and can be caused by an injury or by repetitive strains. Angie was just starting physical therapy but was already concerned about surgery even though many patients with rotator cuff pain don't ever need an operation. Her question made me wonder whether her doctor focused on the eventual need for a surgical repair rather than laying out more conservative approaches that are often effective.

Angie could use the "Know Your Alternatives" portion of the CARES model to understand the "what else?" of rotator cuff syndrome. This would arm her with the information she needs to discuss the full range of treatment options with her doctor.

- "Go to" MayoClinic.org.
- Link to the Patient Care and Health Information section and search "rotator cuff."
- Read the Definition and watch the video to understand the physical abnormality causing shoulder pain.
- The Treatment section provides information about using physical therapy and cortisone injections (as well as surgery) to treat a rotator cuff injury. The Self-Management section explains the steps Angie can take at home (rest, avoiding movements that trigger pain, applying ice and heat, and taking pain relievers). These complement the medical treatment plan, make Angie an active participant in her care, and may help her avoid surgery.

Facebook Question

*Mike: Does a morning cortisol level of 2 (normal range 8–25) automatically mean adrenal insufficiency? What if three consecutive morning cortisol levels were 2.0, 2.2, and 4.0? The symptoms are fatigue, muscle pain, weakness, and more. I did my research on the Cleveland Clinic website and it says that a morning level less than 3.0 confirms the diagnosis.*

*Dr. Georgiou: Consistently low morning cortisol levels are very suggestive of adrenal insufficiency. However, keep in mind that adrenal insufficiency can be caused by a problem with the adrenal gland itself (primary adrenal insufficiency), the pituitary gland (secondary), or the hypothalamus (tertiary). This is not a common condition and requires that a specialist make the diagnosis. Are you seeing an endocrinologist?*

*Mike: This is for my daughter. We were referred to an endocrinologist, but she downplayed the lab results. Then when I asked for a second opinion, she got offended. This is a frustrating process.*

*Dr. Georgiou: You have every right to get a second opinion and don't need to ask her permission. Just make sure you select another endocrinologist who is an expert in adrenal insufficiency.*

Adrenal insufficiency occurs when the body doesn't make enough cortisol, a critical hormone that helps maintain the body's blood pressure, immune response, and metabolism. Mike had clearly researched the condition and understood its implications. While he was asking me to interpret his daughter's laboratory results, what he really wanted and needed was validation that he could *and should* take this daughter to another specialist.

Mike could use the "Know Your Alternatives" and the "Respect Your Preferences" portions of the CARES model to identify an endocrinologist specializing in adrenal insufficiency:

- "Go to" Healthgrades.com.
- In the Hospital tab, search for hospitals in Minneapolis, Minnesota, the city where Mike lives.

- Refine the search to identify hospitals with the best quality outcomes. Because adrenal insufficiency is rare, there are not specific hospital mortality and complications data for this condition. So refine the list by filtering for "America's Best 100 Hospitals Awards" under the Healthgrades Awards category. Three hospitals appeared in the list with one being closest to his home.
- Call the hospital's chief of staff. Ask for his recommendations for endocrinologists specializing in adrenal insufficiency. Ask friends and colleagues for their recommendations. In this scenario, the primary care physician's recommendation is less likely to be helpful because he made the referral to the first specialist. Look for duplicate recommendations. Create a short list of doctors.
- "Go to" Healthgrades.com. Only consider physicians who are board certified in *both* internal medicine and endocrinology. Review malpractice and disciplinary sanctions. Narrow the list further by comparing patient satisfaction results. (Tip: When I am looking for a super-specialist, I frequently take an extra step and read each doctors' biography on their personal website. This gives me an additional glimpse into their expertise and area of focus.)

Facebook Question

*Karen: I have nail fungus on three toes of one foot and am thinking about having those nails removed. What do you think?*

*Dr. Georgiou: Removing the nails can work, but there can be recurrence of the fungal infection or there can be complications. So have you considered all the options? The first is doing nothing since this problem is merely cosmetic. The second is taking oral medications that could treat all your toes. However, it's expensive (since it may not be covered by insurance), may have liver side effects, and takes a long time to work.*

*Karen: Is the oral medication the one that affects the liver?*

Toenail fungus is unattractive but not a condition that even needs treatment. Ironically, the option of doing nothing makes the decision-making process more difficult because doing something could result in serious complications. Because Karen is asking about nail removal, I will assume she already tried some home remedies and over-the-counter antifungal nail creams and ointments to get rid of her nail fungus. Her dilemma was whether to have surgery or take medication.

I didn't answer Karen's question because immediately after posting her question on Facebook, she said she had to sign off and go to work. My response, however, would have encouraged her to make a decision using the concepts from the "Respect Your Preferences" and "Evaluate Your Options" portions of the CARES model:

- Clarify "what matters most." Is the goal to eliminate the toenail fungus so that her feet look attractive in sandals? Or is the goal to eliminate pain and foul odor being caused by the toenails separating from the nail bed? The answer will influence her preferences.
- With surgery, the medical risks are low, but there is short-term impact on her quality of life because her toenails won't grow back for twelve to eighteen months. While there are not long-term complications, surgery only has a 50 percent success rate. The financial commitment is insignificant because the majority of the cost is covered by insurance.
- With oral medication (the most common is terbanifine), the medical risk of liver injury is rare: 1 in 125,000. Short term, the most significant quality-of-life issue is the duration of the treatment (twelve weeks) and the hassle of taking a daily medication. Cure rates average about 75 percent, though it takes up to year to see the full results. Because the medication comes in generic form, the financial commitment is insignificant.
- With or without a cure, the surgery commits her to a long cosmetic recovery. The medication poses a remote risk of liver damage but a higher cure rate without any cosmetic impact. With this information, Karen could decide which approach gives her peace of mind.

Facebook Question

*Melanie: My husband, Joe, has to have both knees and hips replaced, but the doctor says he has to lose weight first. He weighs close to 350 pounds. He's supposed to lose 100 pounds before surgery. He's watching what he's eating, but because of the pain he can't exercise. Consequently, the weight is not coming off. What else can he do?*

*Dr. Georgiou: If your husband needs to lose 100 pounds, then he is unlikely to lose that by "trying to watch what he is eating." He needs to find a program that works for him and then commit to it. Weight Watchers, Jenny Craig, or Nutrisystem are well-known, credible companies that offer the three key components of weight loss: structured food intake, group support, and a system of accountability. Your husband should compare the features, price, locations, etc., of all these programs to decide which is the best for him. And if you are willing, this may be something you could do together since it would be a healthy lifestyle change for both of you.*

I've received hundreds of questions from viewers on diet, nutrition, weight loss, and exercise, but Melanie's question was one of the most serious. At 350 pounds, Joe's morbid obesity was not only preventing him from having surgery, it also made him immobile and put him at risk for blood clots, skin breakdown, infections, and, just as importantly, made him unable to fully participate in his life.

Presumably, Joe understood his condition, considered his alternatives, and decided that he would have four joint replacement surgeries to address his top priority: eliminating arthritis pain in his hips and knees. However, that first step depended on Joe losing weight. Like so many patients, Joe probably walked out of the surgery clinic without a tangible plan to lose the necessary 100 pounds. But he could have used the CARES model, in collaboration with his doctor, to "Start Taking Action" toward his goal:

- What (exactly) could Joe do over the next thirty days? If he'd asked, his doctor may have suggested a nutrition consultation to help him assess weight management programs as well as a series of physical therapy visits to assess his ability to exercise.
- What (exactly) could Joe do over the next sixty days? Assuming Joe stayed engaged with his plan, he would be actively enrolled and participating in a weight management program and committed to sticking to an exercise plan.
- What (exactly) could Joe do over the next ninety days and beyond? He would continue on his plan and keep his doctor informed about his progress and any changes in his symptoms. With

just 10 percent weight loss (thirty-five pounds), Joe would predictably feel less pain and be more mobile.

- With the positive "side effects" from the weight loss, Joe and his doctor could reassess whether he really needs all four joints replaced.
- A log of Joe's progress will help Joe and his surgeon predict when he is likely to meet the one-hundred-pound goal. This lets them create a tentative surgery schedule, which gives Joe and Melanie an opportunity to plan for inpatient stay and recovery.

Each of these viewers needed the partnership of a doctor or provider to achieve their health goal. Jen's husband would ultimately need a sleep study; Angie would need to continue treatment with her physical therapist; Mike needed the expertise of a super-specialist; Karen would need her podiatrist to either do surgery or prescribe medication; and Joe would need the support of a dietician, physical therapist, and his doctor—as well as his wife.

However, these examples show you how Jen, Angie, Mike, Karen, and Joe didn't have to passively wait and wonder about their health. They could use the approaches I've laid out to actively participate in their care, or in the care of someone they love. Jen's research could help her influence her husband to get care, and Angie's could motivate her to stay adherent to her treatment plan in order to avoid surgery. Mike could use the model to help him advocate for his daughter and assure she gets the best care, and Karen's insight into her own priorities could help prevent a decision she might later regret. Joe's targeted questions could accelerate his opportunity to live an active life. When you learn to use the CARES model, it can become a "go to" tool to help you take charge of your health.

# 10

# THE CARES MODEL AT A GLANCE

I've laid out the details about how to use the CARES model to help you make choices regarding medical treatments, complementary and alternative medicine, living arrangements as you age, end-of-life decisions, physicians, and health insurance. This chapter consolidates the key steps so that you have the entire framework of the CARES model at your fingertips.

Five key steps of the CARES model include:

- Understand Your **Condition**: know the "so what?" of your medical situation.
- Know Your **Alternatives**: be informed about "what else" you should consider before making a decision.
- **Respect** Your Preferences: honor "what matters most" and integrate your financial, medical, personal, and quality-of-life values into your decision.
- **Evaluate** Your Options: make the choice that "gives you peace of mind" now and in the future.
- **Start** Taking Action: ask "what's next?" and take responsibility for implementing your decision.

## MAKE MEDICAL TREATMENT DECISIONS USING CARES

"Go to" sites:

- MayoClinic.org
- WebMD.com

Understand Your **Condition** by getting smart about your disease and knowing:

- The symptoms, causes, and risk factors.
- How the condition alters the body's normal function.
- How the condition progresses and threatens your health.
- The signs and symptoms indicating that the condition needs treatment by a medical professional.

Know Your **Alternatives** by researching:

- How your condition affects your treatment options.
- Other treatments that are available.
- The short- and long-term benefits of each treatment.
- The short- and long-term risks of each alternative.
- How to self-manage this condition.

**Respect** Your Preferences by clarifying your values regarding:

- How you want your health to improve as a result of treatment.
- Why the treatment result is important to you.
- Medical risks you are willing to take to improve your health.
- Short-term quality-of-life consequences you are willing to tolerate.
- Long-term quality-of-life consequences you are willing to accept and endure.
- The financial commitment you are willing to make to improve your health.
- The role of your cultural and religious beliefs in your healthcare decisions.

**Evaluate** Your Options and create a bridge to decision making by:

- Eliminating options that do not meet your health goals.
- Setting aside options that pose excessive short- and long-term medical risks.

- Balancing the best outcomes with acceptable quality-of-life trade-offs.
- Identifying the options that you can afford.
- Identifying the options you can choose with peace of mind and without regret.
- Discussing the options with your physician in a meeting that you direct with a clear agenda.

**Start** Taking Action by:

- Creating a calendar to organize the responsibilities you have for your care.
- Being knowledgeable about what to expect during treatment.
- Understanding treatment side effects.
- Establishing rational indicators that the treatment is working, and identifying the point when you'll move on to a new option.

## ASSESS COMPLEMENTARY AND ALTERNATIVE MEDICINE OPTIONS USING CARES

"Go to" sites:

- National Center for Complementary and Integrative Health (nccih.nih.gov)
- Office of Cancer Complementary and Alternative Medicine (cam.cancer.gov)
- Cochrane Complementary Medicine website (cam.cochrane.org)

Understand Your **Condition** by knowing the difference between the biological aspect of the disease and the symptoms:

- List the bothersome symptoms associated with your condition.
- Learn the side effects you are likely to experience as a result of the treatment.
- Be honest with yourself about the symptoms you are most afraid of and how they might disrupt your quality of life.

Know Your **Alternatives** by using credible sources to identify complementary and alternative medicine (CAM) treatments that may treat your symptoms. For each CAM option, research:

- The evidence showing that it works.
- The short- and long-term benefits.
- The short- and long-term risks.
- The conditions under which the treatment is covered by insurance.

**Respect** Your Preferences by considering:

- The complexity of integrating CAM treatments into a conventional medical treatment plan.
- The inconvenience associated with added visits for CAM services.
- The insurance coverage and cost associated with CAM treatments.

**Evaluate** Your Options by weighing your priorities and balancing:

- The importance of eliminating or minimizing the symptoms addressed by CAM options.
- The complexity, inconvenience, and cost trade-offs associated with CAM options.
- The effect of CAM options on conventional medical care alternatives.

**Start** Taking Action by identifying a competent practitioner:

- Call your local hospital or medical school for provider recommendations.
- Understand your state and local government's requirements for licensing and certification of practitioners.
- Verify the licensure status and certification of every provider prior to the initial visit.
- Keep all of your physicians and practitioners well informed about your care plan.

## MAKE DECISIONS AROUND AGING AND END OF LIFE USING CARES

"Go to" sites:

- National Institute on Aging (nia.nih.gov)
- AARP (aarp.org)
- U.S. Living Will Registry (uslivingwillregistry.com)
- Everplans (everplans.com)
- Death over Dinner (http://deathoverdinner.org)
- The Conversation Project (http://theconversationproject.org)

Understand Your **Condition** by knowing that aging may affect your ability to live independently if:

- You become unable to take care of your basic needs.
- You can no longer manage your personal responsibilities.
- Your ability to think and interact diminishes.
- You experience increasing difficulty with moving and walking.

Also understand the medical events that quickly lead to and are commonly present at end of life:

- Your heart stops beating.
- Your lungs stop breathing.
- Your kidneys fail to filter the toxins in your blood.
- An infection invades the bloodstream.
- Malnutrition results in muscle wasting.
- Pain is pervasive and persistent.

Know Your **Alternatives** by considering all your choices about where to live as you age. These include:

- Staying at home or moving in with family, friends, or caregivers.
- A retirement community.
- An independent living community.
- An assisted living community.
- A memory care unit (within an assisted living community).
- A nursing home.

- A continuing care retirement community.

Also know the medical interventions you want to have when you are nearing the end of life:

- Cardiopulmonary resuscitation.
- Ventilator support.
- Kidney dialysis.
- Antibiotics, antiviral, and antifungal medications.
- Feeding tube and intravenous fluids.
- Pain medications.

**Respect** Your Preferences by visualizing yourself on a future day. Imagine the challenges you might face and the accommodations you prefer if you have:

- Difficulty moving and walking.
- Difficulty managing your personal responsibilities or performing basic self-care needs.
- Difficulty interacting with the people around you.

Imagine yourself in a healthy dying experience and your preferences for:

- Personal care and comfort.
- Social support.
- Funeral and memorial plans.
- Medical treatment.
- A healthcare agent who can speak on your behalf if you cannot speak for yourself.

**Evaluate** Your Options by assembling and engaging a team of trusted advisors, including your:

- Spouse/partner.
- Children.
- Other family members.
- Close friends.
- Accountant/financial advisor.

- Lawyer.
- Clergy/spiritual support.
- Physician.

**Start** Taking Action by completing the legal documents that help assure your wishes are met, including:

- Advance directive: *both* a living will and a durable power of attorney for healthcare.
- Durable power of attorney.
- Medical records release.

## SELECT A PHYSICIAN USING CARES

"Go to" sites:

- Healthgrades (Healthgrades.com) for objective physician and hospital data.
- ProPublica's Surgeon Scorecard (propublica.org/data) for physician procedure volumes on selected procedures.

Understand Your **Condition** and navigate toward the right type of specialist by:

- Using a credible health information site to determine your diagnosis, and/or
- Asking your primary care physician to identify the clinical specialty that typically treats your condition.

Know Your **Alternatives** by getting specialist recommendations from:

- The chief of staff at the hospital with the best outcomes for your condition.
- Your primary care physician.
- Your social network.

Narrow the recommendations to the short list of specialists whose names are repeatedly mentioned.

**Respect** Your Preferences by collecting objective information about the specialists you are considering, including their:

- Specialty and subspecialty board certification.
- Practice specialization.
- Malpractice history.
- Disciplinary actions.
- Patient satisfaction.

**Evaluate** Your Options by paying attention to the interpersonal dynamics during an initial face-to-face visit. Think about whether you are comfortable:

- Asking questions.
- Admitting your fears and expressing your preferences.
- Disagreeing with the physician's point of view or recommendation.

Also consider whether you feel the physician:

- Answers questions using words and phrases that you understand.
- Listens and responds to your concerns.
- Respects your opinion and treats you like an equal partner in the relationship.

**Start** Taking Action by arming yourself and your doctors with your complete medical history. Collect your medical records dating back three to five years, and with every new visit ask for your own copy of:

- Laboratory test results.
- Radiology reports.
- EKGs and other diagnostic tests.
- Specialty consultation summaries.
- Operative reports, including results of surgical pathology.


## BUY HEALTH INSURANCE USING CARES

"Go to" sites:

- Healthcare Bluebook (healthcarebluebook.com)

Understand Your **Condition** by analyzing your use of healthcare services:

- Predict the number of office visits, diagnostic tests, inpatient and outpatient admissions, and other healthcare services.
- Make realistic assumptions about potential medical encounters by looking at your pattern of unplanned, urgent, and emergency visits.
- Estimate the cost for each predicted and potential medical encounter.
- Estimate next year's total medical costs.

Know Your **Alternatives** by understanding the basic components of health insurance:

- *Premium:* The amount you pay for insurance during a policy year.
- *Deductible:* The amount you contribute toward your medical costs *before* your insurance company pays for any benefits during a policy year.
- *Copayment:* A specified dollar amount you contribute toward the cost of a service.
- *Coinsurance:* A specified percentage you contribute toward the cost of a specific service.
- *Out-of-Pocket Maximum:* The most you'll have to contribute toward the cost of your medical care during a policy year.
- *Out-of-Network Benefit:* A specified percentage of the allowed amount that your insurance will pay for care from out-of-network providers.

**Respect** Your Preferences by creating your own side-by-side comparison of policy options. Compare plans based on the following trade-offs:

- Financial risk: premium, deductible, copayment, coinsurance, out-of-pocket maximum, and out-of-network benefits.
- Choice: gatekeeper versus open access model for specialist referrals.

- Access: network status of your physicians and the prominent tertiary care/trauma hospitals in your area.
- Coverage: exclusions for specific services that are relevant to you.

**Evaluate** Your Options by calculating your *total* insurance costs for each plan option. For each plan option, enter:

a. Plan monthly premium
b. Plan deductible
c. Plan copayment amounts
d. Plan coinsurance percentage (the lower percentage)
e. Maximum out-of-pocket costs
f. Next year's total medical cost

Then calculate:

g. Annual premium (multiply a x 12)
h. Amount of the deductible that you will pay (insert b or f, whichever is less)
i. Medical costs that exceed your deductible (subtract f – b)
j. Amount of copayments that you will pay*

    * Add together the copayments you'll pay for each visit/encounter

k. Amount of coinsurance that you will pay (multiply d x i)
l. Your cumulative contribution for medical care (add h + j + k)*

    * If the cumulative contribution is more than your maximum out-of-pocket costs (e), replace l with the amount in e because this is the maximum out-of-pocket cost you pay in a premium year.

m. Your TOTAL* cost (add g to l)

    * This combines your cumulative contribution and the insurance premium.

**Start** Taking Action by reading your policy's Summary Plan Description and understanding how your health insurance works before you need to use it. Focus on:

- What's covered.
- What's excluded.

- Your contribution toward the cost of medical services you receive: deductible, copayments, coinsurance, out-of-pocket maximum, and out-of-network benefits.
- The plan's requirements for specialist referrals and prior authorization for hospitalizations and other services.
- Your appeal and grievance rights.

# BIBLIOGRAPHY

AARP. "About Continuing Care Retirement Communities." *AARP.org*. Accessed February 1, 2016. http://www.aarp.org/relationships/caregiving-resource-center/info-09-2010/ho_continuing_care_retirement_communities.html.

Accenture Consulting. "Accenture Consulting Research Report, 2014." Accessed April 4, 2016. https://www.accenture.com/us-en/insight-private-health-insurance-exchange-annual-enrollment.aspx.

ageLoc. "New Anti-Aging Trends." Accessed January 12, 2016. http://www.ageloc.com/content/ageloc/en/anti-aging_trends/market_overviews.html.

American Board of Medical Specialties. *2013–2014 ABMS Board Certification Report*. Accessed March 20, 2016. http://www.abmsdirectory.com/pdf/Resources_certification_statistics.pdf.

American Customer Satisfaction Index. "Benchmarks by Industry." Accessed April 5, 2015. http://www.theacsi.org/customer-satisfaction-benchmarks/benchmarks-by-industry.

America's Health Insurance Plans. "Milliman Report: High-Value Healthcare Provider Networks." July 1, 2014. Accessed April 15, 2014. https://ahip.org/wp-content/uploads/2016/02/High-Value-Provider-Networks-Issue-Paper-2014_07_01.final-pdf.pdf.

Andallu, B., V. Suryakantham, B. L. Srikanthi, and G. K. Reddy. "Effect of Mulberry (*Morus indica* L.) Therapy on Plasma and Erythrocyte Membrane Lipids in Patients with Type 2 Diabetes." *Clinica Chimica Acta International Journal of Clinical Chemistry and Diagnostic Laboratory Medicine* 314 (2001): 47–53.

Archelle MD. https://www.facebook.com/archellemd.

Ashok, M., S. J. Blalock, E. J. Coker-Schwimmer, C. E. Golin, C. D. Jones, K. N. Lohr, D. L. Rosen, P. Sista, M. Viswanathan, and R. C. Wines. "Interventions to Improve Adherence to Self-Administered Medications for Chronic Diseases in the United States: A Systematic Review." *Annals of Internal Medicine* 157 (2012): 785–95.

Assisted Living Federation of America. "2013 Survey of Assisted Living Residents." Accessed February 1, 2016. http://www.alfa.org/Document.asp?DocID=512.

Ball, Mary, Molly M. Perkins, Carole Hollingsworth, Frank J. Whittington, and Sharon V. King. "Pathways to Assisted Living." *Journal of Applied Gerontology* 28, no. 1 (February 2009): 81–108.

Barnes, P. M., Eve Powell-Griner, Kim McFann, PhD, and Richard L. Nahin. "Complementary and Alternative Medicine Use Among Adults and Children: United States, 2007." *National Health Statistics Reports*, no. 18 (July 30, 2009).

Bengoechea, I., Susana Garcia Gutiérrez, Kalliopi Vrotsou, Miren Josune Onaindia, and Jose Maria Quintana Lopez. "Opioid Use at the End of Life and Survival in a Hospital at Home Unit." *Journal of Palliative Medicine* 13, no. 9 (September 2010): 1079–83.

Berman, Brian M., R. Barker Bausell, Susan M. Hartnoll, Mac Beckner, and Joseph Bareta. "Compliance with Requests for Complementary-Alternative Medicine Referrals: A Survey of Primary Care Physicians." *Integrative Medicine* 2, no. 1 (December 1999): 11–17.

Birkmeyer, John D., Therese A. Stukel, Andrea E. Siewers, Philip P. Goodney, David E. Wennberg, and F. Lee Lucas. "Surgeon Volume and Operative Mortality in the United States." *The New England Journal of Medicine* 349 (November 27, 2003): 2117–27, doi:10.1056/NEJMsa035205.

Blendon, R. J. "Understanding the Managed Care Backlash." *Health Affairs*, no. 4 (1998): 80–94.

Board of Health Promotion and Disease Prevention. "Integration of CAM and Conventional Medicine." *Complementary and Alternative Medicine in the United States*. Committee on the Use of Complementary and Alternative Medicine by the American Public. Washington, DC: National Academies Press, 2005.

———. "Prevalence, Cost, and Patterns of CAM Use." *Complementary and Alternative Medicine in the United States*. Committee on the Use of Complementary and Alternative Medicine. Washington, DC: National Academies Press, 2005.

Braddock, Clarence H., K. A. Edwards, N. M. Hasenberg, T. L. Laidley, and W. Levinson. "Informed Decision Making in Outpatient Practice: Time to Get Back to Basics." *Journal of the American Medical Association* 282, no. 24 (December 22, 1999): 2313–20, doi:10.1001/jama.282.24.2313.

Breen, Catherine, Amy P. Abernethy, Katherine H. Abbott, and James A. Tulsky. "Conflict Associated with Decisions to Limit Life-Sustaining Treatment in Intensive Care Units." *Journal of General Internal Medicine* 16, no. 5 (2001): 283–89.

BrideBox. "Women Are Dating Longer Before Getting Engaged." *BrideBox.com*. Accessed February 23, 2016. http://www.bridebox.com/blog/couples-date-before-engagement.

Brown, A. "Evaluating the Reasons Underlying Treatment Nonadherence in VLU Patients: Mishel's Theory of Uncertainty: Part 2 of 2." *Journal of Wound Care* 23, no. 2 (February 2014): 73–80.

Bruera, E. "Patient Preferences Versus Physician Perception of Treatment Decisions in Cancer Care." *Journal of Clinical Oncology* 19, no. 11 (June 1, 2001).

Buettner, Dan. *Blue Zones: Lessons for Living Longer From the People Who've Lived the Longest*. Washington, DC: National Geographic Society, 2008.

Butler, E. Sonny. "Consumers Ranking of Criteria for Selection of a Primary Care Physician, 2002." *International Association for Computer Information Systems*. Accessed February 25, 2016. http://iacis.org/iis/2002/ButlerMcGlone.pdf.

California Health Care Foundation (2005).

Carrns, Ann. "Long-Term Care Costs Rising." *New York Times*, April 9, 2013. Accessed April 27, 2016. http://bucks.blogs.nytimes.com/2013/04/09/long-term-care-costs-rising/.

Castillo, Lesley S., Brie A. Williams, Sarah M. Hooper, Charles P. Sabatino, Lois A. Weithorn, and Rebecca L. Sudore. "Lost in Translation: The Unintended Consequences of Advance Directive Law on Clinical Care." *Annals of Internal Medicine* 154, no. 2 (January 18, 2011): 121–28, doi:10.7326/0003-4819-154-2-201101180-00012.

Cataldo, J. L., J. M. de Godoy, and N. de Barros. "The Use of Compression Stockings for Venous Disorders in Brazil." *Phlebology: The Journal of Venous Disease* 27, no. 1 (2012): 33–37, doi:10.1258/phleb.2011.010088.

Center for Nutrition Advocacy. "State Map of Current Laws." Accessed January 5, 2015. http://www.nutritionadvocacy.org/laws-state.

Centers for Disease Control and Prevention. "Colorectal Cancer Screening Rates Remain Low." November 5, 2013. http://www.cdc.gov/media/releases/2013/p1105-colorectal-cancer-screening.html.

———. "National Center for Health Statistics." http://www.cdc.gov/nchs/fastats/physician-visits.htm.

———. "National Health Interview Survey." January–March 2014. http://www.cdc.gov/nchs/nhis/index.htm.

———. "Prescription Opioid Overdose Data." Accessed April 21, 2016. http://www.cdc.gov/drugoverdose/data/overdose.html.

Centers for Medicare and Medicaid Services. "CMS Finalizes 2016 Medicare Payment Rules for Physicians, Hospitals and Other Providers." October 30, 2015. Accessed February 15, 2016. https://www.cms.gov/Newsroom/MediaReleaseDatabase/Press-releases/2015-Press-releases-items/2015-10-30.html.

———. "National Health Expenditure Projections 2012–2022: Forecast Summary." http://www.cms.gov/Research-Statistics-Data-and-Systems/Statistics-Trends-and-Reports/NationalHealthExpendData/downloads/proj2012.pdf.

———. "NHE Fact Sheet." Accessed April 8, 2016. https://www.cms.gov/research-statistics-data-and-systems/statistics-trends-and-reports/nationalhealthexpenddata/nhe-fact-sheet.html.

Charles, Cathy, Amiram Gafnv, and Tim Whelan. "Shared Decision-Making in the Medical Encounter: What Does It Mean? (Or It Takes At Least Two to Tango)." *Social Science and Medicine* 44, no. 5 (1997): 681–92. http://emed.einstein.yu.edu/auth/pdf/138898.pdf.

Cherry, Donald K., David Woodwell, E. N. Hing, and Elizabeth A. Rechsteiner. "National Ambulatory Medical Care Survey: 2006 Summary." *National Health Statistics Reports*, no. 3 (August 6, 2008). http://www.cdc.gov/nchs/data/nhsr/nhsr003.pdf.

Clarke, Tainya C., Lindsey I. Black, Barbara J. Stussman, Patricia M. Barnes, and Richard L. Nahin. "Trends in the Use of Complementary Health Approaches Among Adults: United States, 2002–2012." *National Health Statistics Reports*, no. 7 (February 10, 2015).

Cordina, Jenny A., Thomas Pellathy, and Shubham Singhal. "The Role of Emotions in Buying Health Insurance." *McKinsey&Company*. Accessed April 19, 2016. http://healthcare.mckinsey.com/sites/default/files/768912_The_role_of_emotions_in_buying_health_insurance.pdf.

Daniels, K., and W. D. Mosher. "Contraceptive Methods Women Have Ever Used: United States, 1982–2010." *National Health Statistics Reports* 62 (February 14, 2013).

Dasenbrock, H. H., M. J. Clarke, T. F. Witham, C. M. Sciubba, Z. L. Gokaslan, and A. Bydon. "The Impact of Provider Volume on the Outcomes After Surgery for Lumbar Spinal Stenosis." *Neurosurgery* 70, no. 6 (June 2012): 1346–54, doi:10.1227/NEU.0b013e318251791a.

Diffen. "HMO vs PPO." Accessed April 16, 2015. http://www.diffen.com/difference/HMO_vs_PPO.

Drug Discovery and Development. "Opioid-Induced Constipation Treatment Market Will Boom to $650M by 2019." Accessed April 21, 2016. http://www.dddmag.com/news/2015/12/opioid-induced-constipation-treatment-market-will-boom-650m-2019.

Engelmann, Jan B., C. Monica Capra, Charles Noussair, and Gregory S. Berns. "Expert Financial Advice Neurobiologically 'Offloads' Financial Decision-Making Under Risk." *Public Library of Science ONE* 4, no. 3 (March 24, 2009), doi:10.1371/journal.pone.0004957.

Evans, M., A. Shaw, E. A. Thompson, S. Falk, P. Turton, T. Thompson, and D. Sharp. "Decisions to Use Complementary and Alternative Medicine (CAM) by Male Cancer Patients: Information-Seeking Roles and Types of Evidence Used." *BMC Complementary Alternative Medicine* 7, no. 25 (August 4, 2007), doi:10.1186/1472-6882-7-25.

Family Caregiver Alliance National Center on Caregiving. Accessed February 1, 2016. https://www.caregiver.org.

Federation of State Medical Boards. *U.S. Medical Regulatory Trends and Actions.* May 2014. Accessed March 20, 2016. https://www.fsmb.org/Media/Default/PDF/FSMB/Publications/us_medical_regulatory_trends_actions.pdf.

Fogg, B. J., Leslie Marable, Julianne Stanford, and Ellen R. Tauber. "How Do Users Evaluate the Credibility of Web Sites? A Study with Over 2,500 Participants." Accessed October 23, 2015. http://htlab.psy.unipd.it/uploads/Pdf/lectures/captology/p1-fogg.pdf.

Freburger, J. K., George M. Holmes, Robert P. Agans, Anne M. Jackman, Jane D. Darter, Andrea S. Wallace, Liana D. Castel, William D. Kalsbeek, and Timothy S. Carey. "The Rising Prevalence of Chronic Low Back Pain." *Archives of Internal Medicine* 169, no. 3 (2009): 251–258, doi:10.1001/archinternmed.2008.543.

Freedman, Vicki A., and Brenda C. Spillman. "Disability and Care Needs of Older Americans: An Analysis of the 2011 National Health and Aging Trends Study." April 11,

2014. Office of the Assistant Secretary for Planning and Evaluation U.S. Department of Health and Human Services.

Frost and Sullivan. "Patient Nonadherence: Tools for Combating Persistence and Compliance Issues." December 2005. Accessed September 21, 2015, www.frost.com/prod/servlet/cpo/115071625.pdfý.

Furlow, M. L., D. A. Patel, A. Sen, and J. R. Liu. "Physician and Patient Attitudes Towards Complementary and Alternative Medicine in Obstetrics and Gynecology." BMC Complementary and Alternative Medicine 8, no. 35 (2008), doi:10.1186/1472-6882-8-35.

Garrido, Melissa M., E. L. Idler, H. Leventhal, and D. Carr. "Pathways from Religion to Advance Care Planning: Beliefs About Control Over Length of Life and End-of-Life Values." The Gerontologist 53, no. 5 (2013): 801–16, doi:10.1093/geront/gns128.

Gavaix, Xavier, and David Laibson. "Shrouded Attributes, Consumer Myopia, and Information Suppression in Competitive Markets." National Bureau of Economic Research. November 2005. Accessed April 10, 2016. http://www.nber.org/papers/w11755.pdf.

Genworth Financial. "Genworth 2015 Cost of Care Survey Home Care Providers, Adult Day Health Care Facilities, Assisted Living Facilities and Nursing Homes." Accessed February 1, 2016. https://www.genworth.com/dam/Americas/US/PDFs/Consumer/corporate/130568_040115_gnw.pdf.

Greene, B. R., M. Smith, V. Allareddy, and M. Haas. "Referral Patterns and Attitudes of Primary Care Physicians Towards Chiropractors." BM Complementary and Alternative Medicine 6, no. 5 (2006): doi:10.1186/1472-6882-6-5.

Greenfield, S., S. H. Kaplan, J. E. Ware, E. M. Yano, and H. J. Frank. "Patients' Participation in Medical Care." Journal of General Internal Medicine 3, no. 5 (1988): 448.

Hamburg, M. E., C. Finkenauer, and C. Schuengel. "Food for Love: The Role of Food Offering in Empathic Emotion Regulation." Frontiers in Psychology 5, no. 32 (January 31, 2014). http://journal.frontiersin.org/article/10.3389/fpsyg.2014.00032/full.

Hanauer, D. A., K. Zheng, D. C. Singer, A. Gebremariam, and M. M. Davis. "Public Awareness, Perception, and Use of Online Physician Rating Sites." The Journal of the American Medical Association 311, no. 7 (2014): 734–35.

Health Affairs. "The New Era of Narrow Networks: Do They Come at the Cost of Quality?" Health Affairs Blog. October 13, 2015. Accessed April 9, 2015. http://healthaffairs.org/blog/2015/10/13/the-new-era-of-narrow-networks-do-they-come-at-the-cost-of-quality/.

———. "Where Is Hitech's $35 Billion Dollar Investment Going?" Health Affairs Blog. Accessed March 28, 2016. http://healthaffairs.org/blog/2015/03/04/where-is-hitechs-35-billion-dollar-investment-going/.

Healthcare Bluebook. Accessed April 9, 2016. https://healthcarebluebook.com.

HealthCare.gov. "10 Health Care Benefits Covered in the Health Insurance Marketplace." HealthCare.gov Blog. Accessed April 16, 2016. https://www.healthcare.gov/blog/10-health-care-benefits-covered-in-the-health-insurance-marketplace/.

HealthDay News. "Most Doctors Not Knowledgeable About Herbals." April 26, 2010. Accessed June 15, 2010. www.modernmedicine.com/modernmedicine/Modern+Medicine+Now/Most-Doctors-Not-Knowledgeable-About-Herbals/ArticleNewsFeed/Article/detail/666928.

Healthgrades. "Healthgrades 2016 Report to the Nation." October 2015. Accessed March 4, 2016. http://www.healthgrades.com/quality/healthgrades-2016-report-to-the-nation.

———. "What Americans Don't Know About Their Doctors and Hospital May Be Putting Their Health at Risk." October 23, 2012. http://www.healthgrades.com/about/press-room/what-americans-dont-know-about-their-doctors-and-hospitals-may-be-putting-their-health-at-risk.

Healthgrades Consumer Survey. Healthgrades.com. Accessed proprietary data 2012. http://www.healthgrades.com/.

Helyer, Lucy K., Stephen Chin, Betty K. Chui, Barbara Fitzgerald, Sunil Verma, Eileen Rakovitch, George Dranitsaris, and Mark Clemons. "The Use of Complementary and Alternative Medicines Among Patients With Locally Advanced Breast Cancer—A Descriptive Study." BMC Cancer 6, no. 39 (February 2006), doi:10.1186/1471-2407-6-39.

Hess, T. M., C. Aumna, S. J. Colcombe, and T. A. Rahhal. "The Impact of Stereotype Threat on Age Differences in Memory Performance." *The Journals of Gerontology: Psychological Sciences* 58, no. 1 (January 2003): P3–11.

Holmes-Rovner, Margaret, Jill Kroll, Neal Schmitt, David R. Rovner, M. Lynn Breer, Marilyn L. Rothert, Georgia Padonu, and Geraldine Talarczyk. "Patient Satisfaction with Health Care Decisions: The Satisfaction with Decision Scale." *Medical Decision Making* 16, no. 1 (January–March 1996): 56–64.

Informed Medical Decisions Foundation. *Informing and Involving Patients in Medical Decisions: The Primary Care Physicians' Perspective* (February 2009). http://informedmedicaldecisions.org/wp-content/uploads/2009/02/PCP_Perspective_WhitePaper.pdf.

Institute for Healthcare Improvement. "Your Conversation Starter Kit: When It Comes to End-of-Life Care, Talking Matters." The Conversation Project and the Institute for Healthcare Improvement, 2015. Accessed February 10, 2016. http://theconversationproject.org/wp-content/uploads/2015/11/TCP_StarterKit_Final.pdf.

Internal Revenue Code of 1939. Pub. L. No. 1, Sec. 104, 76th Cong. (1939).

Internal Revenue Code of 1954. Pub. L. No. 83–591, Sec. 106, 83rd Cong. (1954).

Jena, A. B., S. Seabury, D. Lakdawalla, and A. Chandra. "Malpractice Risk According to Physician Specialty." *The New England Journal of Medicine* 365, no. 7 (2011): 629–36.

Joint Center for Housing Studies. "Housing America's Older Adults—Meeting the Needs of an Aging Population." Harvard University, 2014. Accessed January 27, 2016. http://www.jchs.harvard.edu/sites/jchs.harvard.edu/files/jchs-housing_americas_older_adults_2014.pdf.

Jones, R. M., K. J. Devers, A. J. Kuzel, and S. H. Woolf. "Patient-Reported Barriers to Colorectal Cancer Screening: A Mixed-Methods Analysis." *American Journal of Preventive Medicine* 38, no. 5 (2010): 508–16, doi:10.1016/j.amepre.2010.01.021.

Kaiser Family Foundation. "2016 Employer Health Benefits Survey." September 14, 2016. Accessed November 11, 2016. http://kff.org/health-costs/report/2016-employer-health-benefits-survey/.

———. "Total Professionally Active Physicians." January 2016. Accessed February 24, 2016. http://kff.org/other/state-indicator/total-active-physicians/.

King, N., L. G. Balneaves, G. T. Levin, T. Nguyen, J. G. Nation, C. Card, T. Truant, and L. E. Carlson. "Surveys of Cancer Patients and Cancer Health Care Providers Regarding Complementary Therapy Use, Communication, and Information Needs." *Integrative Cancer Therapies* 14, no. 6 (November 2015): 515–24.

KSTP-TV Channel 5. https://www.facebook.com/KSTPTV.

Kuluski, Kerry, Ashlinder Gill, Gayathri Naganathan, Ross Upshur, R. Liisa Jaakkimainen, and Walter P. Wodchis. "A Qualitative Descriptive Study on the Alignment of Care Goals Between Older Persons with Multi-Morbidities, Their Family Physicians and Informal Caregivers." *BMC Family Practice* 14, no. 133 (2013), doi:1186/1471-2296-14-133.

Kyrrus. "2014 Physician Referral Survey." Accessed March 1, 2016. https://www.kyruus.com/hubfs/Kyruus_Whitepaper_Physician_Referral_Sentiment.pdf?submissionGuid=2366d71e-30d9-4811-bdd8-df1118df813b.

Laine, C., F. Davidoff, C. E. Lewis, E. C. Nelson, E. Nelson, R. C. Kessler, and T. L. Delbanco. "Important Elements of Outpatient Care: A Comparison of Patients' and Physicians' Opinions." *Annals of Internal Medicine* 125, no. 8 (October 15, 1996): 640–45.

Lawlor, D. A., and S. M. Nelson. "Effect of Age on Decisions about the Numbers of Embryos to Transfer in Assisted Conception: A Prospective Study." *The Lancet* 379 (2012): 521.

Lee, C. N., R. Dominik, C. A. Levin, M. J. Barry, C. Cosenza, A. M. O'Connor, A. G. Mulley Jr., and K. R. Sepucha. "Development of Instruments to Measure the Quality of Breast Cancer Treatment Decisions." *Health Expectations* 13, no. 3 (2010).

Leiberic, Peter, Thomas Loew, Karin Tritt, Claas Lahmann, and Marius Nickel. "Body Worlds Exhibition—Visitor Attitudes and Emotions." *Annals of Anatomy* 188, no. 6 (November 14, 2006): 567–73.

Löckenhoff, Corinna E., F. De Fruyt, A. Terracciano, R. R. McCrae, M. De Bolle, P. T. Costa Jr., M. E. Aguilar-Vafaie, C. K. Ahn, H. N. Ahn, L. Alcalay, J. Allik, T. V. Avdeyeva,

C. Barbaranelli, V. Benet-Martinez, M. Blatný, D. Bratko, T. R. Cain, J. T. Crawford, M. P. Lima, E. Ficková, M. Gheorghiu, J. Halberstadt, M. Hrebícková, L. Jussim, W. Klinkosz, G. Knezević, N. L. de Figueroa, T. A. Martin, I. Marusić, K. A. Mastor, D. R. Miramontez, K. Nakazato, F. Nansubuga, V. S. Pramila, A. Realo, J. P. Rolland, J. Rossier, V. Schmidt, A. Sekowski, J. Shakespeare-Finch, Y. Shimonaka, F. Simonetti, J. Siuta, P. B. Smith, B. Szmigielska, L. Wang, M. Yamaguchi, and M. Yik. "Perceptions of Aging Across 26 Cultures and Their Culture-Level Associates." *Psychology and Aging* 24, no. 4 (2009): 941–54, doi:10.1037/a0016901.

Loewenstein, George, Joelle Y. Friedman, Barbara McGill, Sarah Ahmad, Suzanne Linck, Stacey Sinkula, John Beshears, James J. Choi, Jonathan Kolstad, David Laibson, Brigitte C. Madrian, John A. List, and Kelvin G. Volpp. "Consumers' Misunderstanding of Health Insurance." *Journal of Health Economics* 32, no. 5 (September 2013): 850–62.

Luft, H. S., J. P. Bunker, and A. C. Enthoven. "Should Operations Be Regionalized? The Empirical Relation Between Surgical Volume and Mortality." *The New England Journal of Medicine* 301, no. 25 (1979): 1364–69.

Lyons, Imogen. "Public Perceptions of Older People and Ageing—A Literature Review." National Center for the Protection of Older People. November 2009. Accessed January 14, 2016. http://www.ncpop.ie/ncpopresearch_review1.

MacDonald, Jay. "How Bad Is Shopping for Health Insurance?" *Bankrate.com*. Accessed April 12, 2016. http://www.bankrate.com/finance/insurance/health-insurance-poll-1114.aspx#ixzz45ftVhpJH.

Mahler, Heike I. M., and James A. Kulik. "Preferences for Health Care Involvement, Perceived Control and Surgical Recovery: A Prospective Study." *Social Science and Medicine* 31, no. 7 (1990): 743–51.

Market Research.com. http://www.marketresearch.com/Marketdata-Enterprises-Inc-v416/Weight-Loss-Status-Forecast-8016030/.

Marquis, M. S., and S. H. Long. "Trends in Manager Care and Competition, 1993–1997." *Health Affairs* 18, no. 6 (1999): 75–88, doi:10.1377/hlthaff.18.6.75. http://content.healthaffairs.org/content/18/6/75.full.pdf?origin=publication_detail.

Martinez-Carter, Karina. "How the Elderly Are Treated Around the World." *The Week*, July 23, 2013. Accessed January 13, 2016. http://theweek.com/articles/462230/how-elderly-are-treated-around-world.

Maslow, Abraham. "Acquiring Knowledge of a Person As a Task for the Scientist." In *The Psychology of Science: A Reconnaissance*, 15. Chapel Hill, NC: Maurice Bassett Publishing, 2007. https://books.google.com/books?id=3_40fK8PW6QC&q=hammer#v=snippet&q=hammer&f=false.

Matthews, S. C., A. Camacho, P. J. Mills, and J. E. Dimsdale. "The Internet for Medical Information About Cancer: Help or Hindrance?" *Psychosomatics* 44 (2003): 100–103.

Medical Malpractice. "Medical Malpractice Basics." Accessed March 18, 2016. http://www.medicalmalpractice.com/topics/medical-malpractice-basics.

Medicare. "Your Medicare Coverage." *Medicare.gov*. Accessed February 1, 2016. https://www.medicare.gov/coverage/long-term-care.html.

Miller, Leona Miller, Jack Goldstein, and Gary Nicolaisen. "Evaluation of Patients' Knowledge of Diabetes Self-Care." *Diabetes Care* 1, no. 5 (September/October 1978): 275–80.

Mulley, Albert G., Chris Trimble, and Glyn Elwyn. *Patients' Preferences Matter: Stop the Silent Diagnosis*. London: The King's Fund, 2012.

Murray, Elizabeth, Bernard Lo, Lance Pollack, and Martha White. "Clinical Decision-Making: Patients' Preferences and Experiences." *Patient Education and Counseling* 65, no. 2 (February 2007): 189–96.

National Cancer Institute. "Acupuncture-Patient Version (PDQ®) Questions and Answers About Acupuncture." Accessed December 28, 2015. http://www.cancer.gov/about-cancer/treatment/cam/patient/acupuncture-pdq/#link/_53.

———. "Fatigue-Patient Version (PDQ®) Causes of Fatigue in Cancer Patients." Accessed December 19, 2015. http://www.cancer.gov/about-cancer/treatment/side-effects/fatigue/fatigue-pdq#section/_27.

———. "Survival Rates for Ovarian Cancer by Stage." Accessed December 27, 2015. http://www.cancer.org/cancer/ovariancancer/detailedguide/ovarian-cancer-survival-rates.

National Center for Complementary and Integrative Health at the National Institutes of Health. Accessed November 17, 2015. https://nccih.nih.gov/health/cancer/camcancer.htm.

———. "Americans Spent $33.9 Billion Out-of-Pocket on Complementary and Alternative Medicine." Last modified February 20, 2013. https://nccih.nih.gov/news/2009/073009.htm.

———. "Paying for Complementary Health Approaches." Accessed December 28, 2015. https://nccih.nih.gov/health/financial.

National Conference of State Legislatures. "Health Insurance: Premiums and Increases." Accessed April 5, 2015. http://www.ncsl.org/research/health/health-insurance-premiums.aspx.

National Council on Aging. "Inaugural United States of Aging Survey." June 2015. Accessed February 5, 2016. https://www.ncoa.org/news/press-releases/inaugural-united-states-of/.

National Institute on Aging. "End of Life: Helping with Comfort and Care." Accessed January 28, 2016. https://www.nia.nih.gov/health/publication/end-life-helping-comfort-and-care/introduction.

National Institute on Deafness and Other Communication Disorders. "Quick Statistics About Hearing." Accessed January 27, 2016. http://www.nidcd.nih.gov/health/statistics/pages/quick.aspx.

Naturopathic Physicians. Accessed January 5, 2015. http://www.naturopathic.org.

Neuberger, Julia Neuberger. "Do We Need a New Word for Patients?" *British Medical Journal* 318 (June 26, 1999): 1756–58. http://dx.doi.org/10.1136/bmj.318.7200.1756.

Nielsen, Jakob. "How Long Do Users Stay on Web Pages?" *NN/g Nielsen Norman Group*. September 12, 2011. Accessed October 27, 2015. http://www.nngroup.com/articles/how-long-do-users-stay-on-web-pages.

Norton, Mira, Liz Hamel, and Mollyann Brodie. "Accessing Americans' Familiarity with Health Insurance Terms and Concepts." *KFF.org*. November 11, 2014. http://kff.org/health-reform/poll-finding/assessing-americans-familiarity-with-health-insurance-terms-and-concepts/.

Obamacare Facts. "ObamaCare Facts: Facts on the Affordable Care Act." Accessed April 4, 2016. http://obamacarefacts.com/obamacare-facts/.

Ober, Josiah. "An Aristotelian Middle Way Between Deliberation and Independent-Guess Aggregation." Stanford/Princeton Working Papers, September 2009. Accessed March 8, 2016. https://www.princeton.edu/~pswpc/pdfs/ober/090901.pdf.

Orstine, Charles Ornstein. "UnitedHealth to Let Doctors Set Treatments." *Dallas Morning News*, November 8, 1999.

PARTNERS+simons. "Partners+Simons National Healthcare Trust Index Shows Five Times More Americans Trust Their Health Plan Than Congress." October 12, 2015. Accessed April 5, 2015. http://www.marketwired.com/press-release/partnerssimons-national-health-care-trust-index-shows-five-times-more-americans-trust-2062985.htm.

Peek, M. E., S. C. Wilson, R. Gorawara-Bhat, A. Odoms-Young, M. T. Quinn, and M. H. Chin. "Barriers and Facilitators to Shared Decision Making Among African-Americans with Diabetes." *Journal of General Internal Medicine* 24, no. 10 (2009): 1135–39.

PhRMA. "From Hope to Cures: PhRMA's Second Annual Health Survey." http://www.phrma.org/sites/default/files/pdf/Second-Annual-PhRMA-Health-Short.pdf.

Pollack, K. M., D. Morhaim, and M. Williams. "The Public's Perspectives on Advance Directives in Maryland: Implications for State Legislative and Regulatory Policy." *Health Policy* 96, no. 1 (2010): 57–63.

Port, Cynthia L., Ann L. Gruber-Baldini, Lynda Burton, Mona Baumgarten, J. Richard Hebel, Sheryl Itkin Zimmerman, and Jay Magaziner. "Resident Contact with Family and Friends Following Nursing Home Admission." *The Gerontologist* 41, no. 5 (2001): 589–96.

Potter, Ned. "Steve Jobs Biographer Walter Isaacson on the Apple CEO's Polarizing Persona." *ABC News*. October 23, 2011. Accessed August 21, 2015. http://abcnews.go.com/

Technology/steve-jobs-biographer-walter-iacson-apple-ceos-polarizing/story?id=
14789445.

PR Newswire. "New Research: One in Six Car Buyers Skips Test-Drive; Nearly Half Visit
Just One (Or No) Dealership Prior to Purchase." April 15, 2014. Accessed March 25,
2016.    http://www.prnewswire.com/news-releases/new-research-1-in-6-car-buyers-skips-
test-drive-nearly-half-visit-just-one-or-no-dealership-prior-to-purchase-255302891.html.

Prince Market Research. "Clarity 2007: Aging in Place in America." August 20, 2007. Accessed February 1, 2016. http://www.slideshare.net/clarityproducts/clarity-2007-aginig-in-
place-in-america-2836029.

PwC Health Research Institute. "Medical Cost Trend: Behind the Numbers 2016." Accessed
April 8, 2016. http://www.pwc.com/us/en/health-industries/behind-the-numbers/behind-
the-numbers-2016.html

Rao, Jaya K., Lynda A. Anderson, Feng-Chang Lin, and Jeffrey P. Laux. "Completion of
Advance Directives Among U.S. Consumers." American Journal of Preventive Medicine
46, no. 1 (2014): 65–70.

Ritenbaugh, C., L. Penney, L. DeBar, D. Welch, J. Schneider, C. Catlin, A. Firemark, and C.
Elder. "OA16.01. Patients, Physicians, and CAM Providers Regard Communication as
Central for Integrating Conventional and CAM Therapies for Chronic Pain." BMC Com-
plementary and Alternative Medicine 12, S1 (2012), doi: 10.1186/1472-6882-12-S1-O62.

Rosin, Tamara. "Consumers Value Objectivity Over Accuracy When Seeking Medical Information: 8 Findings." Becker's Hospital Review. November 17, 2014. Accessed February
25, 2016. http://www.beckershospitalreview.com/hospital-physician-relationships/consu-
mers-value-objectivity-over-accuracy-when-seeking-medical-information-8-findings.html.

Sabriya, Rice. "Dealing with Online Ratings Often Proves Challenging for Doctors." Modern
Healthcare.    March    1,    2014.    Accessed    February    25,    2016.    http://
www.modernhealthcare.com/article/20140301/MAGAZINE/303019970.

Sagi, A., and N. Friedland. "The Cost of Richness: The Effect of the Size and Diversity of
Decision Sets on Post-Decision Regret." Journal of Personality and Social Psychology 93,
no. 4 (2007).

Santarpia, Lidia, Franco Contaldo, and Fabrizio Pasanisi. "Nutritional Screening and Early
Treatment of Malnutrition in Cancer Patients." Journal of Cachexia, Sarcopenia and
Muscle 2, no. 1 (March 2011): 27–35.

Schneiderman, Eric T. "Asks Major Retailers to Halt Sales of Certain Herbal Supplements
As DNA Tests Fail to Detect Plant Materials Listed on Majority of Products Tested."
Letter to retailers, February 3, 2015. Accessed April 27, 2016. http://www.ag.ny.gov/press-
release/ag-schneiderman-asks-major-retailers-halt-sales-certain-herbal-supplements-dna-
tests.

Schwartz, Barry. Paradox of Choice. New York: HarperCollins, 2007. http://wp.vcu.edu/
univ200choice/wp-content/uploads/sites/5337/2015/01/The-Paradox-of-Choice-Barry-
Schwartz.pdf.

Scullard, Paul, C. Peacock, and P. Davies. "Googling Children's Health: Reliability of Medical Advice on the Internet." Archives of Disease in Childhood 95 (April 6, 2010): 580–82,
doi:10.1136/adc.2009.168856.

SeniorHomes. "Independent Living Community Costs: Facts and Figures." Senio-
rHomes.com. Accessed February 1, 2016. http://www.seniorhomes.com/p/independent-
living-costs/.

Sifferlin, Alexandra. "Why Is the Most Effective Form of Birth Control—the IUD—Also the
One No One Is Using?" Time, June 30, 2014. http://time.com/the-best-form-of-birth-
control-is-the-one-no-one-is-using/.

Small Business Development Center. "Assisted Living Facilities." SBDCNet. Accessed February 1, 2016. http://www.sbdcnet.org/small-business-research-reports/assisted-living-fa-
cilities.

Stacey D., F. Légaré, N. F. Col, C. L. Bennett, M. J. Barry, K. B. Eden, M. Holmes-Rovner,
H. Llewellyn-Thomas, A. Lyddiatt, R. Thomson, L. Trevena, J. H. Wu. "Decision Aids for
People Facing Health Treatment or Screening Decisions." Cochrane Database of System-
atic Reviews 1 (2014), doi:10.1002/14651858.CD001431.pub4.

Steinhauser, Karen E., Nicholas A. Christakis, Elizabeth C. Clipp, Maya McNeilly, Lauren McIntyre, and James A. Tulsky. "Factors Considered Important at the End of Life by Patients, Family, Physicians, and Other Care Providers." *The Journal of the American Medical Association* 284, no. 19 (November 15, 2000): 2476–82, doi:10.1001/jama.284.19.2476.

Stelfox, Henry Thomas, Tejal K. Gandhi, John Orav, and Michael L. Gustafson. "The Relation of Patient Satisfaction with Complaints Against Physicians and Malpractice Lawsuits." *The American Journal of Medicine* 118, no. 10 (October 2005): 1126–33.

Stiff, P. J., L. A. Miller, P. Mumby, K. Kiley, R. Batiste, N. Porter, K. Potocki, M. Volle, S. Lichtenstein, S. Wojtowicz, S. Zakrzewski, A. Toor, and T. Rodriguez. "Patients' Understanding of Disease Status and Treatment Plan at Initial Hematopoietic Stem Cell Transplantation Consultation." *Bone Marrow Transplantation* 37, no. 5 (2006): 479–84.

Stripling, Ashley Mae. "Old Talk: An Examination of Reports of Self-Referential and Ageist Speech Across Adulthood." PhD dissertation abstract, University of Florida, August 2011.

Tasmanian Government Department of Health and Human Services. "An Approach to Healthy Dying in Tasmania: A Policy Framework." October 2014. Accessed February 8, 2016. http://www.dhhs.tas.gov.au/__data/assets/pdf_file/0011/175169/DRAFT_for_comment_V_D_October_Healthy_Dying_Framework_Paper.pdf.

———. "What Is Healthy Dying?" Accessed February 8, 2016. http://www.dhhs.tas.gov.au/__data/assets/pdf_file/0006/96378/Web_Healthy_Dying_info_combined.pdf.

TECH TIMES. http://www.techtimes.com/articles/28986/20150127/meet-atx-101-new-magic-injection-to-get-rid-of-your-double-chin-yes-no-surgery-needed.htm.

The American Congress of Obstetricians and Gynecologists. "No Link Between Moderate Caffeine Consumption and Miscarriage." July 21, 2010. http://www.acog.org/About-ACOG/News-Room/News-Releases/2010/No-Link-Between-Moderate-Caffeine-Consumption-and-Miscarriage.

Tompson, T., J. Benz, J. Agiesta, D. Junius, K. Nguyen, and K. Lowell. "Long-Term Care: Perceptions, Experiences, and Attitudes Among Americans 40 or Older." The Associated Press-NORC Center for Public Affairs Research, April 2013.

Transparency Market Research. "Erectile Dysfunction Drugs Market—Global Industry Analysis, Size, Share, Growth, Trends and Forecast 2013–2019." October 21, 2013. Accessed April 16, 2015. https://globenewswire.com/news-release/2015/04/16/725113/10129251/en/Erectile-Dysfunction-Drugs-Market-is-expected-to-reach-an-estimated-value-of-US-3-4-billion-in-2019-Transparency-Market-Research.html.

Twijnstra, Andries, R. H., Mathijs D. Blikkendaal, Erik W. van Zwet, and Frank W. Jansen. "Clinical Relevance of Conversion Rate and Its Evaluation in Laparoscopic Hysterectomy." *Journal of Minimally Invasive Gynecology* 20, no. 1 (January–February 2013): 64–72.

Ubel, Peter A., Andrea M. Angott, and Brian J. Zikmund-Fisher. "Physicians Recommend Different Treatments for Patients than They Would Choose for Themselves." *Archives of Internal Medicine, JAMA Internal Medicine* 3171, no. 7 (April 11, 2011): 630–34.

United Health Foundation. America's Health Rankings. http://www.americashealthrankings.org/reports/annual#sthash.KDoBQmCr.dpuf.

U.S. Department of Health and Human Services. "National Institutes of Health." Accessed December 1, 2015. http://www.hhs.gov/about/budget/fy2015/budget-in-brief/nih/index.html.

van Uden-Kraan, C. F., C. H. Drossaert, E. Taal, E. R. Seydel, and M. A. van de Laar. "Participation in Online Patient Support Groups Endorses Patients' Empowerment." *Patient Education and Counseling* 74, no. 1 (January 2009): 61–69.

Ventola, C. Lee. "Direct-to-Consumer Pharmaceutical Advertising: Therapeutic or Toxic?" *Pharmacy and Therapeutics* 36, no. 10 (October 2011): 669–84. http://www.ncbi.nlm.nih.gov/pmc/articles/PMC3278148/.

Verhoef, Marja J., Lynda G. Balneaves, Heather S. Boon, and Annette Vroegindewey. "Reasons for and Characteristics Associated with Complementary and Alternative Medicine Use Among Adult Cancer Patients: A Systematic Review." *Integrative Cancer Therapies* 4, no. 4 (December 2005): 274.

Vision Health Initiative. Centers for Disease Control and Prevention. Accessed January 27, 2015. http://www.cdc.gov/visionhealth.

Von Hagens, Gunther. "Gunther von Hagens' Body Worlds: The Original Exhibition of Real Human Bodies." Accessed October 21, 2015. http://www.bodyworlds.com/en/exhibitions/past_exhibitions.html.

Vyas, D., and A. E. Hozain. "Clinical Peer Review in the United States: History, Legal Development and Subsequent Abuse." *World Journal of Gastroenterology* 20, no. 21 (June 7, 2014): 6357–63, doi:10.3748/wjg.v20.i21.6357.

Wahner-Roedler, D. L., Ann Vincent, Peter L. Elkin, Laura L. Loehrer, Stephen S. Cha, and Brent A. Bauer. "Physician Attitudes and Knowledge." *eCAM* 3, no. 4 (2006): 495–501.

Weinman, John, Gibran Yusuf, Robert Berks, Sam Rayner, and Keith J. Petrie. "How Accurate Is Patients' Anatomical Knowledge: A Cross-Sectional, Questionnaire Study of Six Patient Groups and a General Public Sample." *BMC Family Practice* 10, no. 43 (2009): doi:10.1186/1471-2296-10-43.

Weinstein, N. D. "Smokers' Unrealistic Optimism About Their Risk." *Tobacco Control* 14, no. 1 (February 2005): 55–59.

Weymiller, A. J., Victor M. Montori, Lesley A. Jones, Amiram Gafni, Gordon H. Guyatt, Sandra C. Bryant, Teresa J. H. Christianson, Rebecca J. Mullan, and Steven A. Smith. "Helping Patients with Type 2 Diabetes Mellitus Make Treatment Decisions: Statin Choice Randomized Trial." *Archives of Internal Medicine* 167, no. 10 (2007): 1076–82.

Wolfe, Sidney M., Cynthia Williams, and Alex Zaslow. "Public Citizen's Health Research Group Ranking of the Rate of State Medical Boards' Serious Disciplinary Actions, 2009–2011." *Public Citizen*. May 17, 2012. Accessed March 20, 2016. http://www.citizen.org/documents/2034.pdf.

World Values Survey Association. http://www.worldvaluessurvey.org/WVSContents.jsp.

Yahanda, Alexander T., Kelly J. Lafaro, Gaya Spolverato, and Timothy M. Pawlik. "A Systematic Review of the Factors that Patients Use to Choose Their Surgeon." *World Journal of Surgery* 40, no. 1 (January 2016): 45–55.

# INDEX

AARP, 93, 98, 171

advance care planning, 92, 93; advance directives, 107–108; approach to, 105–108; barriers to, 92, 97–98, 102; and physician discussion, 100, 102, 103, 106; websites, 106, 108

Affordable Care Act, 21, 24, 149, 150

aging: and ageism, 90–91; and end of life, 96, 100, 102, 104; and healthcare decision-making, 91; healthy dying, 102–104; and living alternatives, 98–99, 101; perceptions of, 89, 90, 92, 93, 94–95, 97–98, 101; preferences, 101–104; websites, 93, 98. *See also* advance care planning; Blue Zones; CARES Model

American Bar Association, 108

American Medical Association, 11, 129

bias. *See* perceptions

Blendon, Robert, 10

Blue Zones, 2; and Dan Buettner, 2, 3, 13n1; longevity factors, 2, 4, 102. *See also* Ikaria

Body Worlds, 54

Buettner, Dan. *See* Blue Zones

CAM. *See* complementary and alternative medicine

Caplan, Arthur, 38–39

CARES Model, ix, 1, 39, 46–47, 126, 159, 166; and aging, 92–108, 171–173; approach, 12–13, 13; and complementary and alternative medicine, 70, 77–85, 169–170; evaluate your options, 44–45, 63–66, 164, 168–169, 170, 172–173, 174, 176; five steps, x, 39, 159, 167; and health insurance, 139–155, 174–177; know your alternatives, 41–42, 56, 57–58, 59–60, 162–163, 168, 170, 171–172, 173, 175; and medical treatment decisions, 167–169; respect your preferences, 42–44, 60–62, 163, 164, 168, 170, 172, 174, 175–176; selecting physicians using, 116–132, 173–174; start taking action, 45–46, 66–67, 165–166, 169, 170, 173, 174, 176–177; understand your condition, 39–40, 52, 53–57, 57–58, 160–161, 168, 169, 171, 173, 175

Carstens, Susan, 79–80

CDC. *See* Centers for Disease Control

Centers for Disease Control, 5

CIGNA Healthcare, 9, 10, 11, 38–39

Clinton, President William, 11

CNN, x, 3, 3–4

Cochrane Complementary Medicine, 77, 169

complementary and alternative medicine: integration with conventional care, 74,

78–79, 81, 83, 85; perceptions, 70–71, 71–72; physician attitudes, 70, 71, 75–76, 77, 83; risks, 71–72, 72, 81, 82; versus conventional care, 70, 73–74, 76; websites, 76–77. *See also* CARES Model

Dallas Morning News, 11
Death over Dinner, 106, 171
direct to consumer advertising, 23

end of life. *See* aging
Everplans, 108, 171
evidence of coverage. *See* health insurance

Facebook questions: aging, 90; benefit coverage, 22, 150; complementary and alternative medicine, 35, 69, 73, 74; credible health information, 24, 29; end-of-life, 94; fear of procedures, 61, 63; health insurance, 139; medication alternatives, 40, 43; persistent symptoms, 53; physician communication, 19; self-care, 15–16, 164–165; specialty care, 116, 128, 162; treatment alternatives, 41, 51, 160, 163

Greece. *See* Ikaria

*Health Affairs*, 10
Healthcare Blue Book, 141
healthcare culture: find it and fix it, 5, 13, 16–17, 23, 33; historical influences, 18–25; and language, 19–20; media influence, 23–24; pharmaceutical industry influence, 16–17, 55; in the United States, 5, 16–17, 54
healthcare decision-making, 1, 31, 33, 38–39, 58, 59, 66; consumer attitudes, 29, 31–32, 42; shared, 32–33, 45, 64–66; trade-offs, 146–152. *See also* aging; CARES Model; patient-physician relationship; preferences
healthcare system, U.S., ix, 17
Health Care Quality Improvement Act, 119
Healthgrades, 119–120, 124, 126, 163, 173

health information websites, 55–56, 56, 57, 58, 114, 141. *See also* advance care planning; aging; complementary and alternative medicine; health insurance; physicians
health insurance, 21, 22, 155; barriers to selecting, 137–138, 151; covered benefits, 81, 82, 149–152; evidence of coverage, 21, 22, 151–152, 155; financial components, 138, 139, 140, 142–146, 147. *See also* Affordable Care Act; CARES Model
Health Insurance Portability and Accountability Act (HIPAA), 131, 132
Health on the Net, 56
health versus healthcare, 4, 5
HMOs. *See* health insurance; managed care

Ikaria, x, 2, 12, 13; expedition, 2–3; healthcare system, 3–4, 4, 5, 13n2; lifestyle, 2; self-reliance, 4. *See also* Blue Zones
insider tips: ageist communication, 90–91; biased online health information, 58; end-of-life conversations, 106; health insurance cost, 147; insurance benefit coverage, 21, 152; "open access" insurance plans, 149; physician communication, 19–20, 76, 83–84; physician credentials, 125, 126; provider networks, 148; specialist recommendations, 122; understanding your condition, 57
integrative medicine. *See* complementary and alternative medicine

Jobs, Steve, 37
Johns Hopkins, 3, 6, 13, 75

Koop, C. Everett, 45
KSTP-TV, x, 12, 16, 80

managed care, 7, 21–22; gatekeeper model, 10, 149; medical director responsibilities, 9–10, 11, 38, 151; medical necessity, 7, 8, 9, 10, 11, 38, 149; networks, 22, 114, 148. *See also* health insurance

MayoClinic, 56, 160, 168
McGuire, William, 10
medical records, 52, 108, 131–132
MetraHealth, 14n6
My Health Care Wishes Pro, 108

National Center for Complementary and
    Integrative Health, 77, 169
National Geographic. *See* Blue Zones
National Institute on Aging, 2, 93, 98, 171

Office of Cancer Complementary and
    Alternative Medicine, 77, 169
Ornstein, Charles, 11

patient-physician relationship, 18, 19–20,
    22, 52, 83–84, 113, 129–131;
    consumers' priorities, 114–115; in
    healthcare decision-making, 31–33,
    42–43, 46
perceptions, 35, 41; risks of, 35–36, 37;
    types of, 36–37. *See also* aging;
    complementary and alternative
    medicine; physicians
physicians, 120, 125; board certification,
    124–125; chief of staff, 120–122, 123;
    consumers' perception of, 113–114,
    126–127; influence of perceptions, 41,
    43, 58, 75, 148; malpractice history,
    123–124, 126–127; quality of care, 119,
    119–120, 123–128, 126–127;
    relationship with insurers, 9, 10, 12,

21–22, 22, 148; specialists, 116–117,
    118, 122–123, 124–125, 148–149;
    websites, 114, 115, 119–120, 126. *See
    also* CARES Model; patient-physician
    relationship
preferences, 34; in healthcare, 34, 60, 61,
    64. *See also* CARES Model; healthcare
    decision-making
priorities. *See* preferences
ProPublica Surgeon Scorecard, 126, 173

RAND Corporation, 7

second opinions, 129
self-reliance, 5
summary plan description. *See* health
    insurance

Tambakakis, Emmanuel, 3
The Conversation Project, 106, 171
thought traps. *See* perceptions

UnitedHealthcare, 10, 11, 13, 14n6, 22
University of Maryland. *See* Cochrane
    Complementary Medicine
University of Minnesota, ix
U.S. Living Will Registry, 108, 171

WebMD, 55, 56, 168
World Values Survey, 18

# ABOUT THE AUTHOR

**Archelle Georgiou**, MD, was the Chief Medical Officer of United-Healthcare, where she changed the company's policies and eliminated the bureaucratic hassles that managed care companies impose on patients and physicians. Since then she has been a nationally recognized physician and consumer advocate who has been invited to speak in diverse forums such as the World Bank, Royal Danish Embassy, Gallup, Mayo Clinic, Wharton School of Business, and Colgate University. She has a regular health news segment on KSTP-TV in Minneapolis and uses the media to empower consumers to be active participants in their health and healthcare. Archelle is an executive in residence at the University of Minnesota Carlson School of Management.

When she's not writing, talking, or thinking about healthcare, Archelle is a mom to her three daughters. She loves to cook (Mediterranean foods, of course), entertain, and travel with her husband. She lives in Wayzata, Minnesota.